Forensic and Legal Medicine - State of the Art, Practical Applications and New Perspectives

Edited by Roberto Scendoni and Francesco De Micco

Published in London, United Kingdom

Forensic and Legal Medicine - State of the Art, Practical Applications and New Perspectives
http://dx.doi.org/10.5772/intechopen.100988
Edited by Roberto Scendoni and Francesco De Micco

Contributors
Yogesh Pal, Vullikanti Vivek Kumar, Deepak Garg, Neeraj Kumar Verma, Mohammed Hedidi, Muhammad Israr, Murad Ali Rahat, Sumaia Saif, Muzafar Shah, Akhtar Rasool, Fazal Akbar, Shahid Ali, Nimra Ishfaq, Eric O. Aigbogun Jr, Tochukwu Egbobe, Gabriel S. Oladipo, Olufemi G. Omitola, Roberto Scendoni, Francesco De Micco

First published in London, United Kingdom, 2023 by IntechOpen
IntechOpen is the global imprint of INTECHOPEN LIMITED, registered in England and Wales, registration number: 11086078, 5 Princes Gate Court, London, SW7 2QJ, United Kingdom

British Library Cataloguing-in-Publication Data
A catalogue record for this book is available from the British Library

Additional hard and PDF copies can be obtained from orders@intechopen.com

Forensic and Legal Medicine - State of the Art, Practical Applications and New Perspectives
Edited by Roberto Scendoni and Francesco De Micco
p. cm.
Print ISBN 978-1-83768-044-3
Online ISBN 978-1-83768-045-0
eBook (PDF) ISBN 978-1-83768-046-7

Meet the editors

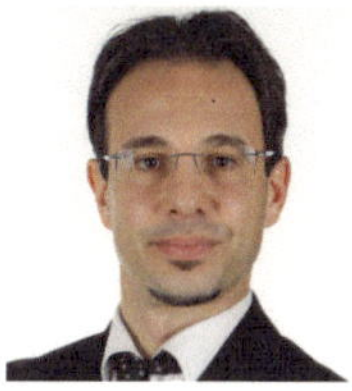

Roberto Scendoni is a medical doctor specializing in legal medicine. In 2022, he received a national scientific qualification as an associate professor in the Italian higher education system of forensic and occupational medicine. He is currently a researcher (MED/43) at the University of Macerata (UniMC), Italy. He is also a consultant for forensic autopsies and external examinations, personal injuries, attempted murders, personal identification, and medical malpractice. His research interests include forensic medicine, forensic anthropology, forensic toxicology, and healthcare management. He has authored/co-authored many journal articles and is an editorial board member for *PLOS One*. Dr. Scendoni has participated in many national and international training events as a speaker and organizer.

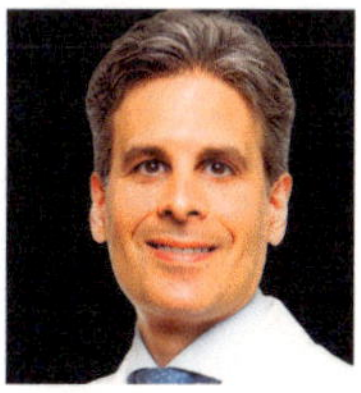

Francesco De Micco is a medical doctor specializing in legal medicine. In 2023, he received a national scientific qualification as an associate professor in the Italian higher education system in forensic and occupational medicine He is currently a researcher in legal medicine (MED/43) at Campus Bio-Medico University, Italy. He is also the clinical risk manager of the Campus Bio-Medico University Hospital Foundation. He conducts research activities in healthcare risk management, forensic medicine, forensic anthropology, and bioethics. He has authored/co-authored many journal articles and is an editorial board member for *PLOS One*. Dr. De Micco has participated in many national and international training events as a speaker and organizer.

Contents

Preface

The term "forensic" has a double meaning. In the most popular sense, forensic science is understood as a particular scientific discipline that is applied to the needs of civil or criminal law. Therefore, an obvious synonym is a legal medicine. In a broader and deeper sense, all the disciplines that can have implications in the judicial field can have a "forensic" terminological connotation. Forensic experts are obliged to explain the smallest details of the methods used, substantiate the choice of the applied technique, and give their unbiased conclusions. Common forensic science disciplines include pathology, anthropology, chemistry, toxicology, nursing, psychiatry, entomology, and engineering. Forensic scientists may be tasked with identifying drugs in the living as well as the deceased and examining molecular biology (DNA), trace evidence, latent fingerprints, firearm and tool marks, handwriting, ballistics and explosives, and computer and digital evidence. Forensic practitioners are often found in laboratories, coroner's offices, universities, or private practices. The introduction of new, sometimes revolutionary, scientific practices is essential for progress in the legal world; in the core pillars of science, and research-based crime prevention and justice systems, forensic teams are a critical component of the law enforcement value chain in support of the timely identification of offenders and their motivations.

This book presents critical and challenging information on certain methods in various disciplines of forensic science.

Roberto Scendoni
Institute of Legal Medicine,
Department of Law,
University of Macerata,
Macerata, Italy

Francesco De Micco
Bioethics and Humanities Research Unit,
Campus Bio-Medico,
University of Rome,
Rome, Italy

Chapter 1

Introductory Chapter: Forensic and Legal Medicine – State of the Art, Practical Applications, and New Perspectives

Roberto Scendoni and Francesco De Micco

1. Introduction

Forensic medicine is a scientific discipline characterized by continuous evolution due not only to advances in medical knowledge but also to changing legal and social needs. On a theoretical level, it is a discipline that contributes to the formation of new laws and the interpretation of existing ones by providing the best scientific evidence. This allows legal norms to be adapted to advances in biological sciences and the social needs of mankind.

From a strictly applicative point of view, forensic medicine using scientific notions has an irreplaceable supporting function for justice.

The perimeter of disciplines pertaining to forensic sciences is progressively expanding. The traditional fields of forensic pathology, forensic anthropology, forensic toxicology, forensic genetics, medical professional responsibility, and bioethics may be complemented and modified by developments in digitalization in healthcare, such as artificial intelligence, virtual reality, and robotics.

The future of forensic science could change radically.

In forensic anthropology, dental age estimation is currently the most widely used method because it is inexpensive and easily applied, and can be applied to both the dead and the living. Age estimation in undocumented individuals undergoing autopsy or in victims of mass disasters are the most common scenarios in which dental age estimation is applied to the dead; in the case of the living, dental age estimation is often used for unaccompanied minors. There are several methods that are based on dental characteristics and development using diagnostic imaging, and their combination allows for increased accuracy of estimation. A multidisciplinary and holistic approach is recommended worldwide, although many health professionals consider medical age assessment, especially when performed through radiology, to be highly invasive and ethically questionable because it is conducted without medical purpose or therapeutic benefit [1–3]. DNA analytical techniques are constantly evolving. In order to offer increasingly reliable tools to investigators, particular attention is being paid to the identification of phenotypic characteristics of the alleged offender [4]. Many authors showed the prospects of the DNA phenotyping technique. With DNA phenotyping, it is possible to predict the phenotypic traits of the alleged offender but also to infer biogeographic ancestry and age estimation using epigenetic markers.

Future studies will presumably lead to increasingly accurate descriptions of a person's appearance from DNA, offering greater value for judicial investigations (homicide, violence, missing persons, etc.).

Emerging/convergent technologies constitute a new field of techno-science characterized by the synergetic integration of several previously separate scientific fields, envisaged as a broad innovation that will lead to a radical modification of mankind and humanity itself. The trends in techno-scientific progress are delineating a new chapter of applied ethics in comparison with the "traditional" topics of biomedical ethics, in the face of which there are composite critical issues emerging, such as the speed of technological evolution, the complexity of technologies, the breadth of applications, the indeterminacy of the traditional boundaries between the medical and nonmedical spheres, the uncertainty related to the lack of data and evidence, and the pervasiveness of technology. The COVID-19 pandemic has greatly increased the use of digital health tools to support communication, information, surveillance, monitoring, and healthcare strategies [5–8]. Some authors demonstrated the development of a new identification models through the integration of artificial intelligence systems and imaging, proceeding to automated image analysis for decision-making-mindedness, and distinguishing in this way positive patients from a negative one [9].

On the other hand, some authors showed the negative implications and threats that can arise from the use of new technologies. Individual behaviors, personality traits, online activities, and attitudes toward technology have an impact on vulnerability. Mental illness can increase vulnerability to cybercrime. In fact, individuals with mental disorders may not be fully aware of the dangers of cybercrime or measures to reduce the risk of certain online behaviors. Cybercrime, so, can promote the transition from virtual sexual aggression to physical sexual aggression. It is, therefore, mandated to develop means to protect people from cyber sexual crimes [10].

In the field of forensic sciences, forensic pathology is an important branch of criminal investigation and has a lot of room for growth with artificial intelligence systems. The traditional way of performing an autopsy and rendering an opinion has many limitations, which can be overcome with machine learning models. Various forensic procedures such as poison analysis, collection of cadaveric biological specimens, detection of pathological changes in the corpse, calculation of post-mortem interval, and detection of a weapon used as a means to injure or kill are the fields where artificial intelligence will play a key role in formulating various judgments of forensic interest [11]. That of forensic autopsies is a minefield, as quality is often questioned [12]; therefore, increasingly innovative and sophisticated approaches will be needed in the near future.

2. Reflection on forensic sciences

Given the nature of the discipline, this book through a multidisciplinary approach aims to offer the reader some reflections on forensic pathology, forensic anthropology, forensic genetics, and the use, positive or negative, of new technologies. Knowing how technological advances can affect this scientific discipline, its criticalities and potential, will enable those who practice it to drive change while always pursuing the protection of the human being.

It is not possible at the moment to predict the technological and scientific discoveries that will shape and advance forensic science in the near future, nor can it be predicted what the footprint will be left by innovative approaches through artificial intelligence systems, but we are convinced that there will be a forensic science based on evidence close to certainty involving the use of highly reliable tools. Investigating the dynamic nature of scientific reconstructions and interpreting the complexity of forensic scientific evidence will be a stimulating challenge.

Author details

Roberto Scendoni[1*] and Francesco De Micco[2]

1 Department of Law, Institute of Legal Medicine, University of Macerata, Macerata, Italy

2 Bioethics and Humanities Research Unit, Campus Bio-Medico University of Rome, Rome, Italy

*Address all correspondence to: scendoni@unimc.it

References

[1] Prince DA, Ubelaker DH. Application of Lamendin's adult dental aging technique to a diverse skeletal sample. Journal of Forensic Sciences. 2002;**47**(1):107-116

[2] Cameriere R, Scendoni R, Ferrante L, Mirtella D, Oncini L, Cingolani M. An effective model for estimating age in unaccompanied minors under the Italian legal system. Healthcare (Basel). 2023;**11**(2):224. DOI: 10.3390/healthcare11020224. PMID: 36673592; PMCID: PMC9859195

[3] De Micco F, Angelakopoulos N, Martino F, Corbi G, Cameriere C, Campobasso CP. Skeletal age estimation in a contemporary South African population using two radiological methods (Bo/Ca and TW2). Australian Journal of Forensic Sciences. 2022;**54**(6):767-784

[4] McCord BR, Gauthier Q, Cho S, Roig MN, Gibson-Daw GC, Young B, et al. Forensic DNA analysis. Analytical Chemistry. 2019;**91**(1):673-688

[5] Cingolani M, Scendoni R, Fedeli P, Cembrani F. Artificial intelligence and digital medicine for integrated home care services in Italy: Opportunities and limits. Frontiers in Public Health. 2023;**10**:1095001. DOI: 10.3389/fpubh.2022.1095001

[6] De Micco F, Fineschi V, Banfi G, Frati P, Oliva A, Travaini GV, et al. From COVID-19 pandemic to patient safety: A new "Spring" for Telemedicine or a Boomerang effect? Frontiers in Medicine (Lausanne). 2022;**15**(9):901788. DOI: 10.3389/fmed.2022.901788

[7] Fedeli P, Scendoni R, Cingolani M, Corrales Compagnucci M, Cirocchi R, Cannovo N. Informed consent and protection of personal data in genetic research on COVID-19. Healthcare (Basel). 2022;**10**(2):349. DOI: 10.3390/healthcare10020349

[8] Travaini GV, Pacchioni F, Bellumore S, Bosia M, De Micco F. Machine learning and criminal justice: A systematic review of advanced methodology for recidivism risk prediction. International Journal of Environmental Research and Public Health. 2022;**19**(17):10594. DOI: 10.3390/ijerph191710594

[9] Pennisi M, Kavasidis I, Spampinato C, et al. An explainable AI system for automated COVID-19 assessment and lesion categorization from CT-scans. Artificial Intelligence in Medicine. 2021;**118**:102114

[10] Monteith S, Bauer M, Alda M, Geddes J, Whybrow PC, Glenn T. Increasing cybercrime since the pandemic: Concerns for psychiatry. Current Psychiatry Reports. 2021;**23**(4):18

[11] Wankhade TD, Ingale SW, Mohite PM, Bankar NJ. Artificial intelligence in forensic medicine and toxicology: The future of forensic medicine. Cureus. 2022;**14**(8):e28376

[12] Scendoni R, Fedeli P, Cannovo N, Cingolani M. The "magnificent seven errors" in forensic autopsy practice: The Italian context. Academic Forensic Pathology. 2021;**11**(4):208-214

Chapter 2

Accuracy and Limits of Lamendin's Age Estimation Method in a Sample of Nigerian Population

Tochukwu Egbobe, Gabriel S. Oladipo,
Olufemi G. Omitola and Eric O. Aigbogun Jr

Abstract

This study compared the accuracy and limits of Lamendin's age estimation method to age estimation by subset regression analysis in a sample of Nigerian population. The research was a cross-sectional study involving 81 single-rooted teeth obtained from 45 females and 36 males between ages 20 and 90 years. Extracted teeth samples were disinfected and stored, and directly measured using a digital vernier caliper on a 16 W X-ray box. Periodontosis (P) and Translucency (T) were derived using standard formulae from the root height (RH), translucency height (TH), and periodontal height (PH). Data were managed in an excel spreadsheet, then analyzed (stratified by sex) using Lamendin's equation (Age = 0.18P + 0.42 T + 25.53) in SPSS (IBM® version 23, Armonk, USA) and Minitab® 2017 (version 18.1) best subset regression for males (Age = 6.23TH + 0.113P + 7.7) and females (Age = 14.90PH + 0.330 T − 2.12). Chi-square analysis tested the distributional deviations from actual age (using error ranges). From the analysis, 33.3% of the total population (M: 30.0% and F: 35.6%) were predicted within the suggested limit compared to 61.7% (M: 75.0% and F: 51.0%) for the best subset model. The distributional errors difference in both methods was not significant for males ($\chi^2_{[df = 3]} = 1.810$, P = 0.405), females ($\chi^2_{[df = 3]} = 1.275$, P = 0.528), and total samples ($\chi^2_{[df = 3]} = 4.960$, P = 0.084). Lamendin's formula did not provide accurate age estimates for a large proportion of sample population. More accurate estimates were limited to age ranged between 30 and 70 years. The study recommended that further studies using a larger sample be conducted to validate the findings of this study.

Keywords: age estimation, Lamendin, best subset, regression, Nigerian population

1. Introduction

Human identification falls under the preview of forensic science, which is simply "the application of science to law" [1]. This means that for forensic science to thrive there must be a legal framework that gives it the spine for functionality, and for the law to truly work, it needs the best practice of forensic science to guide judgment [2]. Unfortunately, this is not globally established. While most developed nations have a legal framework for the practice of forensic sciences, in Nigeria, there is no such law governing forensics, except for the coroner's law that exists in Lagos State, which covers mostly death investigation and not the broader Forensic science application [3]. In the country, there are several lacunae in human identification with little or no database for documentation of such activities.

To solve the puzzles associated with human remains there is the need to determine identity. Therefore, personal identification is necessary for social, legal, and forensic reasons [4]. A massive quest to solve age-related issues about unknown skeletons and living individuals has been on the increase, especially in the field of Forensic Anthropology [5–8]. Matching missing person profiles to biological profiles of unknown remains essential as it provides an informative description for establishing identity. However, this has remained a challenge, especially when there is no comparative information such as dental profile [7, 9].

Over the years, forensic scientists simply match personal information, medical records, and DNA profiling to age [10]. However, in recent times, supplementary methods based on the developing and deteriorating skeleton [11–13], and dental materials [14, 15] have become very useful. Unfortunately, skeletal age indicators are often affected by biological and environmental factors, which vary the rate and degree of age-related changes in the skeleton and can render age estimation inaccurate in adults [16]. Some underlying factors affecting the accuracy of skeletal techniques are high inter- or intra-observer error, higher age ranges, the overlapping of age stages as well as preservation [5, 17]. It is also noted that the discrepancies in age estimation among populations are associated with factors such as economic status, living standards, and pressure of disease, which are known to correlate with age at death [18–20].

In the last 30 years, there has been a significant transformation in forensic odontology, from just occasional dental identification into a wider role, involving building biological profiles [4]. In the living, estimating age in children and adolescents by dental means is usually based on the developmental stages of teeth [21–23], while adults are based on the degenerative changes in teeth like attrition, periodontitis, transparency of the root, secondary dentin, cementum apposition, and root resorption [15, 21, 24–26]. The choice of dental material as an alternative for age estimation becomes necessary when bone-age indicators cannot provide reliable and accurate information [7, 9, 27]. The choice of dental tissues is associated with its self-preserving nature even if the deceased person is skeletonized, decomposed, burnt, or dismembered [28–30]. Thus, dental parameters have become a reliable alternative tool for estimation of sex, age, and ethnicity [19, 31–33].

In 1994, Kvaal and Solheim developed a method for estimating the chronological age of adults based on the relationship between age and the pulp size on periapical dental radiographs [34]. Kvaal et al. method was established by indirectly measuring secondary dentin deposition on radiographs and a number of length and width measurements of teeth and pulp was also proposed. In the Kvaal method, the pulp-to-tooth ratio was calculated using six mandibular and maxillary teeth. They included the maxillary second premolars; maxillary central and lateral incisors; mandibular canine; mandibular lateral incisor; and the first premolar.

Using the pulp-to-tooth ARs in the formula for age determination, age was derived. Using intraoral periapical radiographs, the variables r = complete pulp length/complete tooth length, P = complete pulp length/root length (from enamel-cementum junction [ECJ] to root apex), a = complete pulp length/root width at ECJ level, b = pulp/root width at midpoint level between ECJ level and mid-root level, and c = pulp/root width at the mid-root level and pulp/tooth AR for all six teeth were measured as designed in Kvaal's and Cameriere's methods of age estimation, respectively [34, 35]. Lastly, a simple linear regression analysis was employed, wherein the variables mean (M) (mean of variables complete pulp length/root length [from ECJ to root apex] [p], complete pulp length/complete tooth length [r], complete pulp length/ root width at ECJ level [a], pulp/root width at midpoint level between ECJ level and mid-root level [b], and pulp/root width at mid-root level [c]) and the difference between width and length (W − L) were found to contribute significantly to the chronological age estimation and were utilized in the regression equation for Kvaal's method as per the given formula: Age = 129.8 − (316.4 × M) (6.8 × [W − L]). Other Authors like Bosmans et al. [36], Landa et al. [37], and Li et al. [38] used measurements made on a panoramic radiograph instead of periapical radiographs used in the original formula of Kvaal's technique, thus avoiding the cumbersome full mouth radiographs.

Harris and Nortje and Van Heerden evaluated the mesial root of the third molar for age estimation. They argued that eruption of permanent dentition completes by the age of 17 years, after which it becomes problematic to estimate age from dental radiographs age [39, 40]. One major guide to ascertain the age of an individual after such age is through the examination of the development of the third molar. The Harris and Nortje, and Van Heerden methods involve five stages of third molar root development with corresponding mean ages and mean length: the stages include: Stage 1—cleft rapidly enlarging (one-third root formed); Stage 2—half root formed; Stage 3—two-third root formed; Stage 4—diverging root canal walls; and Stage 5—converging root canal walls [41].

Gustafson in 1947 and 1950 first established a technique for age estimation based on the assessment of certain regressive alterations in teeth. This method is mostly employed on single-rooted teeth using histomorphological approaches [24]. Six age-related parameters; attrition (A), secondary dentin formation (S), periodontal recession (P), cementum apposition (C), root resorption (R), and root transparency (T) were macroscopically assessed using the formula: $A_n + P_n + S_n + C_n + R_n + T_n$ = points (0, 1, 2, 3), and found significant correlations [24]. Gustafson deduced that estimating age using these six criteria appeared equally accurate and effective and that the rates at which the individual criteria change are equal, prompting the addition or summation of the obtained data [42–44]. Gustafson's method has had a major impact on the field of forensic odontology, particular with regards to dental age estimation in adults [45, 46]. Ever since, several studies have considered dental translucency as an important age indicator, making it a pivot for various studies [7, 46–49].

Lamendin et al.'s technique utilize two of the characteristics described by Gustafson [24]; however, his technique is less destructive, uses only one single-rooted tooth, and requires no special technical instrument [50, 51]. Lamendin et al. reduced the number of variables by using root height, periodontal recession, and root transparency, and index values based on actual physical measurements made from the labial aspect of the tooth, then applied a multiple regression analysis to develop his equation which was suitable for both sexes. Lamendin's regression formula for age assessment is as follows: A (age) = (0.18 × P) + (0.42 × T) + 25.53; where P = periodontal height × 100/root height, T = translucency height × 100/root height [46]. In the study, they investigated the accuracy of the method on 306 single-rooted teeth of European (French) and African Ancestry origin, and 45 teeth from 24 forensic cases. The result yielded a mean error of 10 years on their working sample and 8.4 years on their forensic control sample. Furthermore, the application of this data set on individuals below age 40 and above age 70 decreased in accuracy, suggesting cautious use of the method for ages below 40 and above 70 years [46].

Prince and Ubelaker [52] modified Lamendin's method of age assessment. Their new regression formulas incorporated root height (RH) into the equation and calculated the variables "P" and "T" in the same manner as Lamendin et al. [46]. The study results from this modification indicated that age estimation was improved when ancestry and sex of the individual are considered. The formulae was given as

Male African Ancestry: Age= 1.04 (RH) +0.31(P) +0.47(T) + 1.70 =4.97 years
Male European Ancestry: Age =15 (RH) + 0.29(P) + 0.39 (T) +23.17 =5.92 years
Female African Ancestry: Age =1.63 (RH) + 0.48(P) + 0.48 (T) + (−8.41) =7.17 years
Female European Ancestry: Age =1.10 (RH) + 0.39(T) +11.82= 6.21 years

The results of this investigation verified this technique and produced a mean error of 8.23 years and a standard deviation of 6.87 years when Lamendin's formula was utilized. Accuracy was best observed between the chronologic ages of 30 and 69. Higher error rates were observed in subjects younger than 30 and older than 69 years of age [52].

A disadvantage of Lamendin's method is its inapplicability in young individuals (since root translucency occurs from the age of 20) but provides acceptable confidence ranges in adults over the age of 30 [50, 53, 54]. This is argued as one of the benefits of the methods over skeletal age estimation methods which lose their accuracy in adults past age 30 [50, 51]. In a separate study of the accuracy of Lamendin's technique on French autopsy sample of individuals of known age at death, Baccino et al. [51] found that the method produced more accurate estimates than some methods such as estimating age from ribs [55–57], the pubic symphysis [58], and long bone cortical histology [59].

2. Study rationale

Since age estimation is a fundamental requirement in biological profiling of the living and dead; this study opens the basis for the development of national database for different accurate age estimation techniques for the Nigerian population. This study would aid in identifying mutilated bodies of a victim and estimating the age of dead persons in cases of mass disaster. In anthropological studies/research, knowledge of age will assist in the designation of age to Cadavers without anti-mortem information as seen in some gross anatomy labs across Nigerian Universities.

Although there is no legal framework for forensic investigation in Nigeria, this study would provide the impetus for the inclusion of dental methods in solving criminal cases, immigration, and juvenile law enforcement. This will ensure that all legal procedures to which an individual's age is relevant can be properly attained.

Lamedine's age estimation remains the most popular and applied dental age estimation technique, however, there have been a varied degree of accuracy in age estimation using Lamendin's method for different populations [5, 12, 28, 52–54, 60–64]. While in other studies it provided valid and accurate estimates [54, 61, 62], in others the results were described as significantly poor [5, 12, 28, 52, 53, 60, 63, 64]. This study, therefore, comparatively evaluates the accuracy and limits of Lamendin's age estimation method in a sample of the Nigerian Population.

3. Materials and methods

3.1 Study design and protocol

The study research adopted a cross-sectional retrospective research design, which involved the use of dental (teeth) samples obtained from the odontology department of hospitals within the South East and Middle Belt Regions of Nigeria between the months of June 2020 to March 2021. Before carrying out the study, ethical approval with reference numbers UPH/R and D/REC/283 and informed consent were obtained from the University of Port Harcourt Research Ethics Committee and the individual dental centers, respectively. The departments also issued consent forms for the individuals whose samples were included in the study, thus, the pool from which teeth samples were collected had a special number associated with the signed consent.

Dental centers that gave consent to participate in the study collected samples from patients referred for essential clinical care such as periodontal, periapical, orthodontic, and prosthesis construction reasons within the duration of the 3-month study period. The study excluded persons who reported mobile tooth due to trauma and fractured tooth, teeth affected by caries, abscess, root resorption, and abrasion or other pathological processes causing exposure of the root to the oral environment, and teeth presenting any alteration in the root apex, such as ankylosis. The study included all the cases involving dental extraction procedures done as part of essential dental care for permanent teeth, males and females of Nigerian origin, single-rooted maxillary and mandibular teeth, extracted tooth with complete root, and the absence of any pathological conditions in the cervical margin of the tooth or dental restorations. They obtained the following medical information; sex, date, and reason for extraction, and age of the subject at extraction.

Extracted teeth were rinsed in running water and any attached tissue to the root was removed using a pair of tweezers and scalpel. The tooth was then disinfected in 3% hydrogen peroxide (H_2O_2) [11], which is a proven dental health hygiene therapeutic agent which break down dental plaque and calculus, clean gingival tissues, and eliminate bacteria without altering the dental formation [65, 66]. Each tooth was closed in separate small plastic tubes filled with normal saline at 4°C [67] to avoid alteration of the mineral concentration of the tooth surfaces, as demineralization interferes with root translucency (RT).

3.2 Data collection and measurements

The dental measurements were taken using a pair of digital vernier calipers by direct observation with a 16 W X-ray box (**Figure 1**). The measurements were made on the labial surface of the extracted tooth without any preparations (no sections, no microscope).

The study obtained a total of 81 single-rooted permanent teeth (maxillary and mandibular) from the dental centers. The teeth sample comprised of 45 females and 36 males of ages 20–90 years. The root height (RH) is the distance between the apex of the root and the cementoenamel junction, measured on the surface (labial) toward the lips [46, 64, 68]. The periodontal height (PH) which is used to describe the gingival tissue degeneration [46, 61, 64] is obtained from the periodontitis, which is the yellowish area that is darker than the enamel, but lighter than the rest of the root [46, 61], and it is the maximum distance from the cementoenamel junction to the line

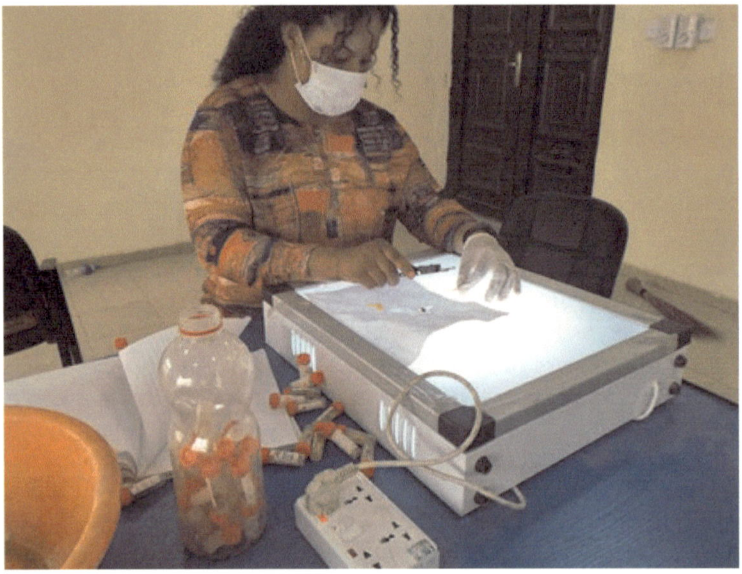

Figure 1.
Light box-aided collection data from stored teeth samples.

left by the soft tissue attachment on the neck and/or root of the tooth. The translucency height (TH) is traditionally measured manually and it is identified as the length of the transparent zone extending from the junction between the translucent and opaque areas of the root to the tip of the root [46, 69]. That is, the distance between the apex of the root and the cementoenamel junction, measured on the surface (labial) toward the lips (**Figure 2**). The indices were derived using the formulae: $P\ (\text{Periodontosis}) = \frac{PH}{RH} \times 100$ and $T\ (\text{Translucency}) = \frac{TH}{RH} \times 100$ were derived [46].

To assess inter-observer error, two independent observers collected the data twice—on different occasions. Inter-observer precision was determined by comparing the results obtained by the two observers. The study compared the average of both measurements for inter-observer reliability.

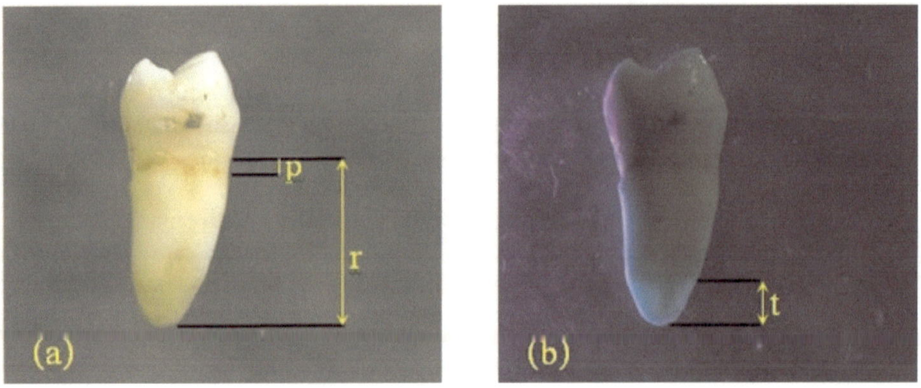

Figure 2.
Measurement of (a) periodontal height (p; PH) and root height (r; RH), (b) translucency height (t; TH) [61].

3.3 Statistical analysis

The measurements were entered into an excel spreadsheet and organized, then imported into Statistical Package for Social Sciences (IBM® version 23, Armonk, USA) and Minitab® 2017 (version 18.1) for statistical analysis. To determine inter-observer precision, paired sample t-test evaluated differences in measurements between the two observers. Lamendin's formula was inputted into SPSS and used to estimate age. The set of variables with the most accurate age estimation combinations was determined using Minitab best subset regression, which was used for the regression model. The study employed the Real statistics [70, 71]—directed scatterplot to determine the relationship between the actual age and the estimates from both methods, and the extent of agreement of the two measurements of both methods using Bland–Altman plot [70].

4. Results

The mean age for the male sample was 35.28 ± 20.84 years, while for females the mean age was 41.42 ± 20.89 years. The ratios; periodontitis (P) and translucency (T) entered into Lamendin's equation for age estimation were derived from the linear dimensions. The measurements from both observers yielded a high inter-observer correlation (r) of 0.980, 0.979, and 0.998 for RH, PH, and TH, respectively (**Table A1**).

To determine how well a regression model would estimate age; using both the linear dimensions and ratios, best subset regression was used to build a model that provided a list of the estimates (RH, PH, TH, P, and T), prediction accuracy and regression for variables (single and multiple; **Tables A2** and **A3**). The regression model built for males in **Table A2** yielded low estimate for age using the dental parameters (linear dimensions and ratios). However, the chosen (observed best) estimate was j2, which had an adjusted accuracy of 53.3% and a predicted accuracy of 48.8%. The parameters that produced this model summary were TH (transparency height) + P (periodontosis). The regression model for females that produced the most accurate estimate was g2; with an adjusted accuracy of 51.2% and a prediction accuracy of 46.6%. The parameters that produced this model summary were PH (periodontal height) + T (translucency) (**Tables A3**).

In **Table 1**, the age estimation error differences for Lamendin's method (A [age in years] = 0.18P + 0.42 T + 25.53) and the best subset regression for males (A [age in years] = 6.23 TH + 0.113 P + 7.7) were compared, and there was underestimation using Lamendin's method for males starting at age greater than 40 years, then at age 56 using best subset regression; however, larger estimate error was found in the best subset (age 90; at ±52 and ± 43) when compared to Lamendin's estimate (±50 and ± 45) for the same age. For females, the outcome of the calculations from the regression equation for age estimation using Lamendin's method (A [age in years] = 0.18P + 0.42 T + 25.53) and the best subset regression equation (A [age in years] = 14.90 PH + 0.330 T − 2.12) were compared. The result indicated a constant negative error difference (−actual age) started at age 44 using Lamendin's formulae, but age 28 for the best subset. A larger estimate error for age was found in Lamendin's estimate (±35 to ±42) when compared to the best subset (age 90; at ±23 to ±27) for different ages (**Table 2**).

The distribution of the estimates with the error margin using the Lamendin's range of ≤ ± 10 years obtained from both methods revealed that only about 33.3% of the

Sex	Actual age	Lamedine's Estimation A (age in years) = 0.18P + 0.42 T + 25.53	*d1*	Regression (from Subset) A (age in years) = 6.23 TH + 0.113 P + 7.7	*d2*
M1	20	33	13	24	4
M2	20	35	15	28	8
M3	21	37	16	30	9
M4	21	36	15	29	8
M5	21	37	16	32	11
M6	22	36	14	23	1
M7	22	41	19	39	17
M8	23	36	13	28	5
M9	23	37	14	30	7
M10	24	35	11	23	−1
M11	24	37	13	27	3
M12	25	35	10	27	2
M13	25	35	10	25	0
M14	25	34	9	22	−3
M15	25	35	10	22	−3
M16	25	36	11	27	2
M17	26	38	12	28	2
M18	26	33	7	19	−7
M19	26	40	14	32	6
M20	26	38	12	27	1
M21	27	35	8	23	−4
M22	27	39	12	27	0
M23	27	39	12	33	6
M24	27	39	12	29	2
M25	28	45	17	39	11
M26	30	36	6	32	2
M27	40	58	18	56	16
M28	40	47	7	51	11
M29	56	49	−7	57	1
M30	56	48	−8	56	0
M31	57	55	−2	51	−6
M32	61	41	−20	40	−21
M33	80	57	−23	93	13
M34	80	47	−33	70	−10
M35	90	40	−50	38	−52
M36	90	45	−45	47	−43

Table 1.
Error differences in the estimated age of males using Lamendin's method and best subset regression equation.

Sex	Actual Age	Lamedine's Estimation A (age in years) = 0.18P + 0.42 T + 25.53	*d1*	Regression (from Subset) A (age in years) = 14.90 PH + 0.330 T − 2.12	*d2*
F1	20	32	12	18	−2
F2	20	33	13	31	11
F3	20	38	18	34	14
F4	21	35	14	32	11
F5	21	40	19	29	8
F6	22	38	16	34	12
F7	22	36	14	30	8
F8	23	46	23	44	21
F9	23	49	26	43	20
F10	24	59	35	48	24
F11	24	51	27	41	17
F12	25	37	12	24	−1
F13	25	36	11	32	7
F14	25	38	13	43	18
F15	26	40	14	32	6
F16	27	35	8	31	4
F17	28	42	14	38	10
F18	29	47	18	48	19
F19	30	39	9	30	0
F20	28	36	8	23	−5
F21	29	41	12	44	15
F22	30	36	6	24	−6
F23	34	43	9	31	−3
F24	36	48	12	43	7
F25	36	44	8	31	−5
F26	38	55	17	48	10
F27	42	47	5	35	−7
F28	44	42	−2	27	−17
F29	48	48	0	52	4
F30	49	46	−3	25	−24
F31	50	32	−18	38	−12
F32	50	51	1	57	7
F33	51	44	−7	54	3
F34	53	44	−9	32	−21
F35	55	51	−4	37	−18
F36	56	43	−13	34	−22
F37	56	40	−16	32	−24

Sex	Actual Age	Lamedine's Estimation A (age in years) = 0.18P + 0.42 T + 25.53	*d1*	Regression (from Subset) A (age in years) = 14.90 PH + 0.330 T − 2.12	*d2*
F38	57	65	8	56	−1
F39	66	51	−15	63	−3
F40	75	74	−1	85	10
F41	83	45	−38	56	−27
F42	83	51	−32	60	−23
F43	83	47	−36	56	−27
F44	90	48	−42	77	−13
F45	90	73	−17	82	−8

Table 2.
Error differences in the estimated age of females using Lamendin's method and the regression equation obtained from the best subset.

Variables	Error difference (approximated range) and distribution			χ^2 (*P*-value)
	±1 to ± 10 (%)	±11 to ± 20 (%)	> ± 20 (%)	
Lamendin's method				
Male	11 (30.6)	21 (58.3)	4 (11.1)	1.275 (0.528)
Female	16 (35.6)	21 (46.7)	8 (17.8)	
Total	27 (33.3)	42 (51.9)	12 (14.8)	
Best subset method				
Male	27 (75.0)	6 (16.7)	3 (8.3)	4.960 (0.084)
Female	23 (51.1)	13 (28.9)	9 (20.0)	
Total	50 (61.7)	19 (23.5)	12 (14.8)	

Table 3.
Sex-associated distributional differences in error margins for the estimations using Lamendin's formula and best subset regression.

total population (M: 30.0% and F: 35.6%) fell within the error margin for Lamendin's method and 61.7% (M: 75.0% and F: 51.0%) for best subset regression. The extent of deviation from the actual age ranges for the group ±11 to ±20 years was 51.9% (42 samples) and 23.5% (19 samples) for Lamendin's method and best subset regression, respectively. For the > ± 20 years range, there were equal sample deviations for both Lamendin's method and best subset; 12 samples (14.8%). The difference in the range of sample error in males and females was not significantly different for both methods (Lamendin; χ^2 = 1.275, P = 0.528 and best subset; χ^2 = 4.960, P = 0.084; **Table 3**).

The differences in the proportion of the ranges (error estimate) using both techniques significant for male samples ($\chi^2_{[df = 3]}$ = 15.213, P = 0.0005) and the total samples ($\chi^2_{[df = 3]}$ = 15.542, P = 0.0004) but not females ($\chi^2_{[df = 3]}$ = 3.198, P = 0.202) (**Table 4**). The age ranges 20–24 years, 25–29 years, 30–70 years, and > 30 years were populated and observed for proportion of the Lamendin's estimates that fell within the limit (±10 years). The result showed that age 30–70 years for both males (71.4%) and

Variables	Error difference (approximated range) and distribution			χ^2 (*P*-value)
	±1 to ± 10 (%)	±11 to ± 20 (%)	> ± 20 (%)	
Male				
Lamendin's method	11 (30.6)	21 (58.3)	4 (11.1)	15.213 (0.0005)
Best subset method	27 (75.0)	6 (16.7)	3 (8.3)	
Female				
Lamendin's method	16 (35.6)	21 (46.7)	8 (17.8)	3.198 (0.202)
Best subset method	23 (51.1)	13 (28.9)	9 (20.0)	
Total				
Lamendin's method	27 (33.3)	42 (51.9)	12 (14.8)	15.542 (0.0004)
Best subset method	50 (61.7)	19 (23.5)	12 (14.8)	

Table 4.
Comparison of the distribution of the error differences between Lamendin's methods and best subset regression.

	Limit (±10 years)			
Sex	Age group	within (%)	outside (%)	Total (%)
Male	20–24 years	0 (0)	11 (100)	11 (30.6)
	25–29 years	6 (42.9)	8 (57.1)	14 (38.9)
	30–70 years	5 (71.4)	2 (28.6)	7 (19.4)
	>70 years	0 (0)	4 (100)	4 (11.1)
Female	20–24 years	0 (0)	11 (100)	11 (24.4)
	25–29 years	2 (22.2)	7 (77.8)	9 (20.0)
	30–70 years	13 (68.4)	6 (31.6)	19 (42.2)
	>70 years	1 (16.7)	5 (83.3)	6 (13.3)
Total		27 (33.3)	54 (66.7)	81

Table 5.
Lamendin's estimation using the ±10 years error margin.

females (68.4%); however, lower proportion of the general sample fell within the range (33.3%) (**Table 5**).

The accuracies of the methods are presented in **Figure 3**, while the extent of agreement (Bland–Altman plot) between the two measurements was presented in **Figure 4**. The Scatterplot with regression analysis of the estimated ages using both methods indicated a lower accuracy (R^2) 12.96% for Lamendin's methods when compared to best subset regression (42.62%) (**Figure 3**). The mean difference (bias) for both measures was 3.85 (−12.64 and 20.35 for the lower and upper limits, respectively), and several values were found close to and outside the upper and lower agreement limits (±2SD), which is an indication of discordance in estimates. This was evident as the difference in population mean was statistically significant (t = 3.45; P = 0.001; **Figure 5**).

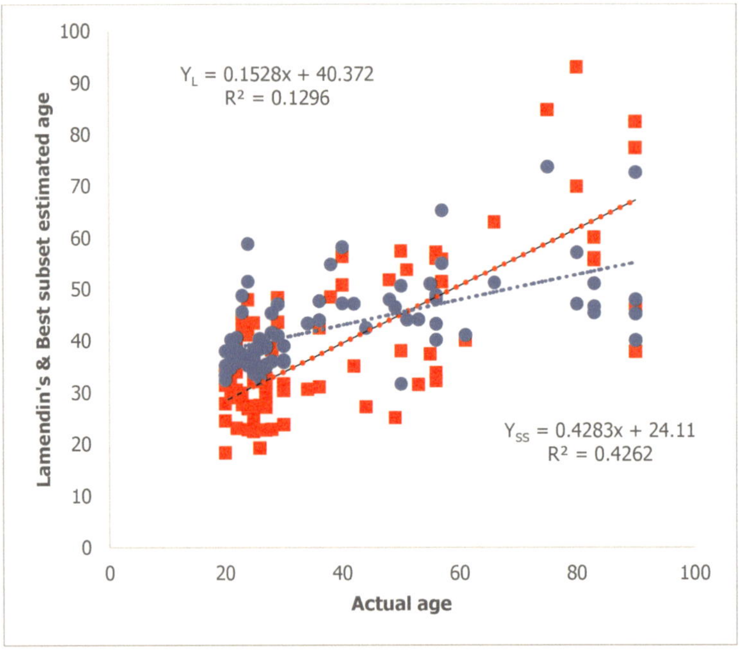

Figure 3.
Scatterplot with regression analysis of Lamendin's (Y_L; blue); best subset (Y_{SS}; red) estimated ages versus Actual age.

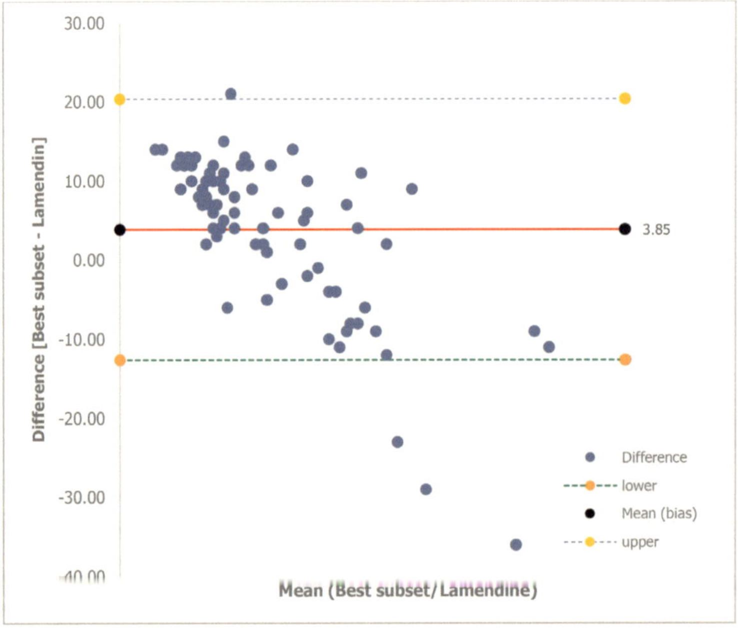

Figure 4.
Bland–Altman plot of the measurement agreement between best subset and Lamendin's method.

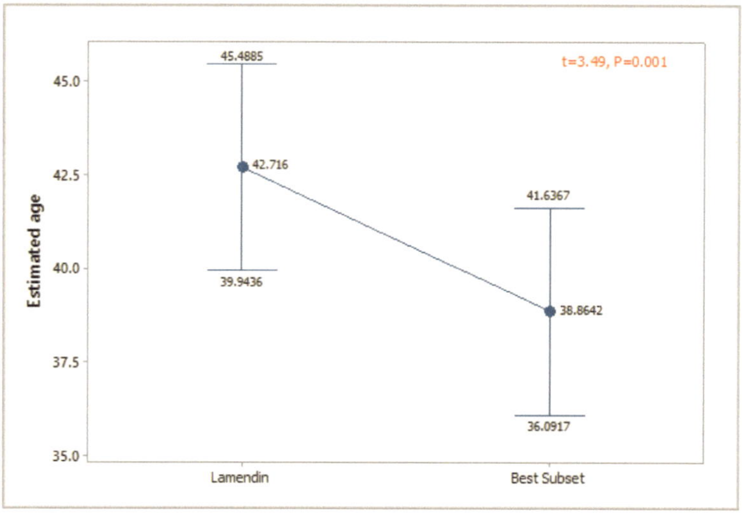

Figure 5.
Interval plot of the mean age prediction for Lamendin's and best subset methods.

5. Discussion

Accuracy and precision are the most important criteria for accepting an age estimation method [50]. This study evaluated the accuracy Lamendin's age estimation method and compared the outcome to that of best subset regression analysis. Although Lamendin et al. (1992) reported unsuitable age estimates for young adults, some studies reported narrower mean error for the estimate [61].

The results for the estimated age using Lamendin's method revealed a wide range of deviations from the error limit ($\pm$10 years) of about $\pm$11 to $\pm$20 (51.9%), $\geq \pm$ 21 (14.8%), with 33.3% falling with the $\pm$10 years age range. The distributional differences for males and females were not significant; however, best subset regression produced more estimates that fell within the error limits for males and the general population compared to Lamendin's method. The original research by Lamendin et al. (1992) which analyzed 306 single-rooted teeth aged 22–90 years, of European Ancestry (French), and African Ancestry proposed that an error of $\pm$10 was obtained, however, 66.7% of the study sample fell outside of this error margin. Garizoain et al. [48] and De Angelis [60] reported wide error ranges of 11.88–15.37, and 10.7–36.8 years, respectively, using Lamendin's method. Wide error margins in age estimation methods have been reported in several studies [5, 12, 28, 52, 53, 60, 63, 64].

When the results from Lamendin's estimates were compared to the best subset regression analysis, the margin of error decreased using the best subset; thus, suggesting a poor age estimation by Lamendin's method in the studied population. Nevertheless, some studies found accurate age estimation using Lamendin's formula [5, 28, 61, 63, 72, 73] and improvement in accuracy and variation when the population had individuals between 40 and 45 years, suggesting that the technique for this age group was very efficient [5, 28, 61–63]. Other studies found more estimates with smaller error margins in groups over 50 years of age [12, 52, 74]. Additional studies have yielded poor age estimation using Lamendin's formulae compared to indigenously derived formulae [63, 75].

According to Prince and Ubelaker [52], Lamendin's method yielded the most accurate age estimates for the 30–69-year-old age groups, which is consistent with Lamendin's original study and the Terry Collection sample. In this study, Lamendin's method did not give predictions lower than age 30 and greater than 74 years. In an attempt to further investigate the age limits for accurate estimates using Lamendin's method, the study restricted the age range to ≥25 years and we found that a more accurate estimate (within ±10 years) was between age 30 and 70 years. The tendency to overestimate age in young adults and underestimate it in older ones is well-documented [6, 48, 49, 60]. Prince and Ubelaker [52] found that when samples were below ages 30 and above 70 years, the mean errors significantly increases. The study also noted differences in error estimates at different age ranges with regard to sex and ancestry, suggesting sex and ancestry could have influenced the age estimation. Previous studies found that sex and ancestry influence error estimate margins [52, 64], but a recent study by Garizoain et al. [48] reported that sex had no influence in age estimation.

The study compared the estimates from both methods and found larger proportions of age estimates outside the previously reported error margin by Lamendin's method; however, the differences in the distribution of the error margins were not significant for males, females, and the total populations. In comparing the accuracy of the actual age to estimates of both methods, the accuracy (R^2) of the estimated age using Lamendin's methods and the best subset were 12.96% and 42.62%, respectively, thus, indicating a poor estimate for the study population using Lamendin's methods and wide difference in age estimates for both methods.

6. Conclusion

With only about 33.3% of the sample age estimated within the error limits, it could be concluded that Lamendin's formula was not accurate for estimating the age in the studied sample of the Nigerian population. The observation of Prince and Ubelaker on the age range (30–70 years) for accurate estimate holds true, as found in our population. The study noted that the regression analysis considered ages 80–90 years as outliers and this could be because of static dentine translucency at this age range.

The study, therefore, recommends further studies using larger sample size from both heterogenous and homogenous populations of Nigerian descent, and that samples that are below 25 years and above 70 years may be excluded, as this study found high proportion of over-estimation for ages below 25 years, and under-estimation for samples above age 70.

6.1 Study limitation

The study noted with concern the difficulty in obtaining single-rooted teeth which significantly reduced the sample population. The uneven distribution of the age of the dental samples posed a concern to the researcher.

There are often more stressful logistics challenges associated with approvals from dental clinics to use their facilities and collection and preservation of samples than carrying out the actual dental measurement. Often times one would be required to wait for weeks before approvals are given and samples are available.

Appendices

Pairs	Variable	Paired differences		Paired sample *t*-test			Paired samples correlations		
		N	MD ± SD	*df*	*t*-value	*P*-value	Pair	*r*	*P*-value
Pair 1 (OB_1–OB_2)	RH_1–RH_2	81	−0.076 ± 0.43	80	−1.622	0.109	RH_1 and RH_2	0.986	<0.001
Pair 2 (OB_1–OB_2)	PH_1–PH_2	81	−0.006 ± 0.15	80	−0.352	0.726	PH_1 and PH_2	0.979	<0.001
Pair 3 (OB_1–OB_2)	TH_1–TH_2	81	0.022 ± 0.18	80	1.096	0.276	TH_1 and TH_2	0.998	<0.001

OB, observer; RH, root height; PH, periodontal height; TH, translucency height; N, distribution; MD, mean difference; SD, standard deviation; df, *degree of freedom;* r, *correlation.*

Table A1.
Inter-observer measurement difference (error) and correlation (precision).

Vars		R^2	R^2 (adj)	R^2 (pred)	Mallows Cp	S	RH	PH	TH	P	T
a	1	55.9	54.6	50.3	−1.0	14.1			X		
b	1	43.3	41.6	34.4	7.9	15.9					X
c	1	10.7	8.1	0	30.8	20.0	X				
e	1	6.1	3.3	0	34.0	20.5				X	
f	1	2.3	0	0	36.7	20.9		X			
g	2	56.2	53.6	45.6	0.8	14.2			X		X
h	2	56.2	53.6	46.7	0.8	14.2		X	X		
i	2	56.1	53.4	48	0.9	14.2	X		X		
j	2	56	53.3	48.8	1.0	14.3			X	X	
k	2	53	50.2	44.6	3.0	14.7	X				X
l	3	56.6	52.5	43.7	2.5	14.4		X	X	X	
m	3	56.5	52.5	41.9	2.6	14.4		X	X		X
n	3	56.4	52.3	43.4	2.6	14.4			X	X	X
o	3	56.4	52.3	44.3	2.7	14.4	X	X	X		
p	3	56.3	52.2	45.4	2.7	14.4	X		X	X	
q	4	56.9	51.3	34.3	4.3	14.6	X	X	X	X	
r	4	56.6	51	37.1	4.5	14.6		X	X	X	X
s	4	56.6	51	36.4	4.5	14.6	X	X	X		X
t	4	56.4	50.8	37.6	4.6	14.6	X		X	X	X
u	4	53.3	47.2	31.4	6.9	15.2	X	X		X	X
v	5	57.3	50.2	25.6	6.0	14.7	X	X	X	X	X

RH, root height; PH, periodontal height; TH, translucency height; P, periodontosis; T, translucency.

Table A2.
Best subset regression analysis for age estimation for males using the measured dimensions and derived indices.

	Vars	R^2	R^2 (adj)	R^2 (pred)	Mallows Cp	S	RH	PH	TH	P	T
a	1	43.5	42.2	38.1	7.5	16.0		X			
b	1	35.6	34.1	29.1	14.3	17.1				X	
c	1	26.6	24.9	20.5	22	18.3					X
e	1	21.6	19.7	13.2	26.4	18.9			X		
f	1	1.1	0	0	43.9	21.2	X				
g	2	53.4	51.2	46.6	1	14.7		X			X
h	2	53.2	51	46.4	1.2	14.7			X	X	
i	2	52.7	50.4	46.3	1.6	14.8		X	X		
j	2	48.7	46.3	39.7	5	15.4				X	X
k	2	47.6	45.1	40.3	6	15.6	X			X	
l	3	54.5	51.1	45.3	2.1	14.7	X		X	X	
m	3	54.4	51	44.7	2.2	14.7	X			X	X
n	3	54.1	50.8	45.6	2.4	14.8		X	X	X	
o	3	54	50.7	43.9	2.5	14.8			X	X	X
p	3	53.6	50.3	44.8	2.8	14.9	X	X	X		
q	4	54.6	50	42.1	4	14.9	X	X	X	X	
r	4	54.5	49.9	41.6	4.1	14.9	X	X		X	X
s	4	54.5	49.9	41.7	4.1	14.9	X		X	X	X
t	4	54.2	49.6	40.9	4.3	15.0		X	X	X	X
u	4	53.7	49	41.9	4.8	15.0	X	X	X		X
v	5	54.6	48.8	37	6	15.1	X	X	X	X	X

RH, root height; PH, periodontal height; TH, translucency height; P, periodontosis; T, translucency.

Table A3.
Best subset regression analysis for age estimation for females using the measured dimensions and derived indices.

Author details

Tochukwu Egbobe[1], Gabriel S. Oladipo[1], Olufemi G. Omitola[2] and Eric O. Aigbogun Jr[3*]

1 Faculty of Basic Medical Sciences, Department of Anatomy, College of Health Science, University of Port Harcourt, Rivers State, Nigeria

2 Faculty of Dentistry, Department of Oral Pathology and Oral Biology, University of Port Harcourt Teaching Hospital, Port Harcourt, Rivers State, Nigeria

3 Faculty of Basic Medical Sciences, Department of Human Anatomy, Enugu State University College of Medicine, Parklane, Enugu, Nigeria

*Address all correspondence to: aigbogun@uniport.edu.ng

References

[1] Jayewardene CHS. Forensic science and the law. Forensic Science International. 1988;**36**(1–2):41-45. DOI: 10.1016/0379-0738(88)90213-7

[2] Eyewu-Edero A. Forensic science and the law. Vanguard New. 2020. Available from: https://www.vanguardngr.com/2020/02/forensic-science-and-the-law/ [Accessed: October 9, 2022]

[3] Law Nigeria Admin. Coroner's system law of Lagos State. Law Nigeria. 2019. Available from: https://laws.lawnigeria.com/2019/04/03/coroners-system-law-of-lagos-state/ [Accessed: October 12, 2022]

[4] Adserias-Garriga J, Thomas C, Ubelaker DH, Zapico SC. When forensic odontology met biochemistry: Multidisciplinary approach in forensic human identification. Archives of Oral Biology. 2018;**87**:7-14. DOI: 10.1016/J.ARCHORALBIO.2017.12.001

[5] Prince DA, Konigsberg LW. New formulae for estimating age-at-death in the Balkans utilizing Lamendin's dental technique and Bayesian analysis. Journal of Forensic Sciences. 2008;**53**(3):578-587. DOI: 10.1111/j.1556-4029.2008.00713.x

[6] Cappella A, Cummaudo M, Arrigoni E, Collini F, Cattaneo C. The issue of age estimation in a modern skeletal population: Are even the more modern current aging methods satisfactory for the elderly? Journal of Forensic Sciences. 2017;**62**(1):12-17. DOI: 10.1111/1556-4029.13220

[7] Stavrianos C, Mastagas D, Stavrianou I, Karaiskou O. Dental age estimation of adults: A review of methods and principals. Research Journal of Medical Sciences. 2008;**2**(5):258-268

[8] Willems G, Moulin-Romsee C, Solheim T. Non-destructive dental-age calculation methods in adults: Intra- and inter-observer effects. Forensic Science International. 2002;**126**(3):221-226. DOI: 10.1016/S0379-0738(02)00081-6

[9] Hillson S. Dental Anthropology. Cambridge University Press; 1996. DOI: 10.1017/cbo9781139170697

[10] Meer Z, Meer A. Modern tools in forensic dentistry. IJCD. 2011;**2**:28-32

[11] Brkic H, Milicevic M, Petrovecki M. Age estimation methods using anthropological parameters on human teeth (A0736). Forensic Science International. 2006;**162**(1–3):13-16. DOI: 10.1016/j.forsciint.2006.06.022

[12] Martrille L, Ubelaker DH, Cattaneo C, Seguret F, Tremblay M, Baccino E. Comparison of four skeletal methods for the estimation of age at death on white and black adults. Journal of Forensic Sciences. 2007;**52**(2):302-307. DOI: 10.1111/j.1556-4029.2006.00367.x

[13] Hartnett KM. Analysis of age-at-death estimation using data from a new, modern autopsy sample—Part II: Sternal end of the fourth rib. Journal of Forensic Sciences. 2010;**55**(5):1152-1156. DOI: 10.1111/j.1556-4029.2010.01415.x

[14] Byers SN. Introduction to Forensic Anthropology. Pearson Education; 2011. Available from: https://books.google.co.ug/books?id=wPKkcQAACAAJ

[15] Adserias-Garriga J, Zapico S. Age assessment in forensic cases: Anthropological, odontological and biochemical methods for age estimation in the dead. Mathews Journal of Forensic Research. 2018;**1**(1):1

[16] Zorba E, Vanna V, Moraitis K. Sexual dimorphism of root length on a Greek population sample. HOMO-Journal of Comparative Human Biology. 2014;**65**(2):143-154. DOI: 10.1016/j.jchb.2013.09.005

[17] Cunha E et al. The problem of aging human remains and living individuals: A review. Forensic Science International. 2009;**193**(1–3):1-13. DOI: 10.1016/j.forsciint.2009.09.008

[18] Puranik M, Uma SR. Dental age estimation methods: A review. 2015; **2016**

[19] Amasiatu VC, Oladipo GS, Oyakhire MO, Aigbogun EO. Estimating the sex of igbo adults using occlusal tooth wear. International Journal of Research and Review. 2019;**6**(8). Available from: www.ijrrjournal.com

[20] Loum Janani KE, Henry K. International Journal of Research and Review. 2015;**2**(6):343-347. Available from: http://www.gkpublication.in/IJRR_Vol.2_Issue6_June2015/IJRR0066.pdf

[21] Cameriere R, Ferrante L, Cingolani M. Age estimation in children by measurement of open apices in teeth. International Journal of Legal Medicine. 2006;**120**(1):49-53. DOI: 10.1007/s00414-005-0047-9

[22] Shumaker DB. A comparison of chronologic age and physiologic age as predictors of tooth eruption. American Journal of Orthodontics. 1974;**66**(1):50-57. DOI: 10.1016/0002-9416(74)90192-4

[23] Moorrees CFA, Fanning EA, Hunt EE. Age variation of formation stages for ten permanent teeth. Journal of Dental Research. 1963;**42**(6):1490-1502. DOI: 10.1177/00220345630420062701

[24] Gustafson G. Age determination on teeth. Journal of the American Dental Association (1939). 1950;**41**(1):45-54. DOI: 10.14219/jada.archive.1950.0132

[25] Hou Y x et al. Dental age estimation using degenerative changes in lower premolars in a northern Chinese population. Rechtsmedizin. 2019;**29**(5):407-414. DOI: 10.1007/s00194-019-00346-3

[26] Parra RC, Ubelaker DH, Adserias-Garriga J, Escalante-Flórez KJ, Condori LA, Buisktra JE. Root dentin translucency and international dental database: Forensic methodology for estimation age-at-death in adults using single-rooted teeth. Forensic Science International. 2020:110572. DOI: 10.1016/j.forsciint.2020.110572

[27] Christensen AM, Passalacqua NV, Bartelink EJ. Forensic Anthropology: Current Methods and Practice. Elsevier Inc.; 2014. DOI: 10.1016/C2013-0-09760-5

[28] Foti B, Adalian P, Signoli M, Ardagna Y, Dutour O, Leonetti G. Limits of the Lamendin method in age determination. Forensic Science International. 2001;**122**(2–3):101-106. DOI: 10.1016/S0379-0738(01)00472-8

[29] Ibeachu C, Aigbogun E. Palatal rugoscopic estimation of sex among Igbo students in the University of Port Harcourt. European Journal of Biomedical and Pharmaceutical Sciences. 2017;**4**(9):58-64. Available from: www.ejbps.com58

[30] Ibeachu C, Aigbogun E, Didia B, Fawehinmi H. Determination of sexual dimorphism by odontometric study using discriminant function analysis of adult ikwerre dental cast. Scholars Journal of Applied Medical Sciences. 2016;**3**:1732-1738. Available from: www.saspublisher.com

[31] Díaz E et al. Frequency and variability of dental morphology in deciduous and permanent dentition of a Nasa indigenous group in the municipality of Morales, Cauca, Colombia. Colombia Médica. 2014;**45**(1):15-24. DOI: 10.25100/cm.v45i1.1281

[32] Moreno-Gomez F. Sexual dimorphism in human teeth from dental morphology and dimensions: A dental anthropology viewpoint. In: Sexual Dimorphism. 2013. DOI: 10.5772/55881

[33] Uthaman C, Sequeira P, Jain J. Ethnic variation of selected dental traits in Coorg. Journal of Forensic Dental Sciences. 2015;7(3):180. DOI: 10.4103/0975-1475.172422

[34] Kvaal S, Solheim T. A non-destructive dental method for age estimation. The Journal of Forensic Odonto-Stomatology. 1994;**12**(1):6-11. Available from: https://pubmed.ncbi.nlm.nih.gov/9227083/ [Accessed: October 12, 2022]

[35] Rösing FW, Kvaal SI. Dental age in adults—A review of estimation methods. In: Dental Anthropology. 1998. pp. 443-468. DOI: 10.1007/978-3-7091-7496-8_22

[36] Bosmans N, Ann P, Aly M, Willems G. The application of Kvaal's dental age calculation technique on panoramic dental radiographs. Forensic Science International. 2005;**153**(2–3):208-212. DOI: 10.1016/j.forsciint.2004.08.017

[37] Landa MI, Garamendi PM, Botella MC, Alemán I. Application of the method of Kvaal et al. to digital orthopantomograms. International Journal of Legal Medicine. 2009;**123**(2):123-128. DOI: 10.1007/s00414-008-0268-9

[38] Li MJ, Chu G, Han MQ, Chen T, Zhou H, Guo YC. Application of the Kvaal method for age estimation using digital panoramic radiography of Chinese individuals. Forensic Science International. 2019;**301**:76-81. DOI: 10.1016/j.forsciint.2019.05.015

[39] Harris MJP, Nortjé CJ. The mesial root of the third mandibular molar. The Journal of Forensic Odonto-Stomatology. 1984;**2**(2):39-43

[40] Heerden V. The mesial root of the third mandibular molar as a possible indicator of age. London: Hospital Medical College; 1985

[41] Nayyar AS, Anand Babu B, Krishnaveni B, Vaishnavi Devi M, Gayitri HC. Age estimation: Current state and research challenges. Journal of Medical Sciences. 2016;**36**(6):209. DOI: 10.4103/1011-4564.196348

[42] Maples WR. An improved technique using dental histology for estimation of adult age. Journal of Forensic Sciences. 1978;**23**(4):10735J. DOI: 10.1520/jfs10735j

[43] Drusini A, Volpe A, Dovigo S. Age determination in human adults by dental histology. Zeitschrift für Morphologie und Anthropologie. 1990;**78**(2):169-174. DOI: 10.1127/zma/78/1990/169

[44] Johanson G. Age determination in human teeth. Odontologisk Revy. 1971;**22**(21):40-126. Available from: https://cir.nii.ac.jp/crid/1571698599600352384 [Accessed: October 12, 2022]

[45] de las Heras SM. Dental age estimation in adults. In: Age Estimation: A Multidisciplinary Approach. 2019. pp. 125-142. DOI: 10.1016/B978-0-12-814491-6.00009-1

[46] Lamendin H, Baccino E, Humbert JF, Tavernier JC, Nossintchouk RM, Zerilli A. A simple technique for age

estimation in adult corpses: The two criteria dental method. Journal of Forensic Sciences. 1992;**37**(5):13327J. DOI: 10.1520/jfs13327j

[47] Solheim T. Dental root translucency as an indicator of age. European Journal of Oral Sciences. 1989;**97**(3):189-197. DOI: 10.1111/j.1600-0722.1989.tb01602.x

[48] Garizoain G, Petrone S, Plischuk M, Inda AM, Garcia MN. Evaluation of Lamendin's age-at-death estimation method in a documented osteological collection (La Plata, Argentina). Forensic Science International: Reports. 2020;**2**:100060. DOI: 10.1016/j.fsir.2020.100060

[49] Sengupta A, Whittaker DK, Shellis RP. Difficulties in estimating age using root dentine translucency in human teeth of varying antiquity. Archives of Oral Biology. 1999;**44**(11):889-899. DOI: 10.1016/S0003-9969(99)00087-4

[50] Soomer H, Ranta H, Lincoln MJ, Penttila A, Leibur E. Reliability and validity of eight dental age estimation methods for adults. Journal of Forensic Sciences. 2003;**48**(1):2002253. DOI: 10.1520/jfs2002253

[51] Baccino E, Ubelaker DH, Hayek L-AC, Zerilli A. Evaluation of seven methods of estimating age at death from mature human skeletal remains. Journal of Forensic Sciences. 1999;**44**(5):12019J. DOI: 10.1520/jfs12019j

[52] Prince DA, Ubelaker DH. Application of Lamendin's adult dental aging technique to a diverse skeletal sample. Journal of Forensic Sciences. 2002;**47**(1):107-116. DOI: 10.1520/jfs15209j

[53] González-Colmenares G, Botella-López MC, Moreno-Rueda G, Fernández-Cardenete JR. Age estimation by a dental method: A comparison of Lamendin's and Prince & Ubelaker's technique. Journal of Forensic Sciences. 2007;**52**(5):1156-1160. DOI: 10.1111/j.1556-4029.2007.00508.x

[54] Zorba E, Goutas N, Spiliopoulou C, Moraitis K. An evaluation of dental methods by Lamendin and Prince and Ubelaker for estimation of adult age in a sample of modern Greeks. Homo. 2018;**69**(1–2):17-28. DOI: 10.1016/j.jchb.2018.03.006

[55] Işcan MY, Loth SR, Wright RK. Age estimation from the rib by phase analysis: White females. Journal of Forensic Sciences. 1985;**30**(3):853-863

[56] Işcan MY, Loth SR, Wright RK. Age estimation from the rib by phase analysis: White males. Journal of Forensic Sciences. 1984;**29**(4):1094-1104

[57] Işcan MY, Loth SR, Wright RK. Racial variation in the sternal extremity of the rib and its effect on age determination. Journal of Forensic Sciences. 1987;**32**(2):452-466

[58] Brooks S, Suchey JM. Skeletal age determination based on the os pubis: A comparison of the Acsádi-Nemeskéri and Suchey-Brooks methods. Human Evolution. 1990;**5**(3):227-238. DOI: 10.1007/BF02437238

[59] Kerley ER. Microscopic determination of age in human bone. American Journal of Physical Anthropology. 1965;**22**:149-163

[60] De Angelis D, Mele E, Gibelli D, Merelli V, Spagnoli L, Cattaneo C. The applicability of the lamendin method to skeletal remains buried for a 16-year period: A cautionary note. Journal of

Forensic Sciences. 2015;**60**(s1): S177-S181. DOI: 10.1111/1556-4029.12611

[61] Lopes JR, Queiroz SBB d S, Fernandes MM, De Paiva LAS, De Oliveira RN. Age estimation by teeth periodontosis and transparency: Accuracy of Lamendin's method on a Brazilian sample. Brazilian Journal of Oral Science. 2014;**13**(1):17-21. DOI: 10.1590/1677-3225v13n1a04

[62] Ribeiro J, Paulo S, Paulo S. Systematic review of Lamendin's dental age estimation method. 2016;**21**(2): 99-109

[63] Meinl A, Huber CD, Tangl S, Gruber GM, Teschler-Nicola M, Watzek G. Comparison of the validity of three dental methods for the estimation of age at death. Forensic Science International. 2008;**178**(2–3):96-105. DOI: 10.1016/j.forsciint.2008.02.008

[64] Ackermann A, Steyn M. A test of the Lamendin method of age estimation in South African canines. Forensic Science International. 2014;**236**:192.e1-192.e6. DOI: 10.1016/j.forsciint.2013.12.023

[65] Inside Dentistry. 3% hydrogen peroxide gel. Inside Dentistry. 2016;**12** (9). Available from: https://www.aegisdentalnetwork.com/id/2016/09/3-hydrogen-peroxide-gel [Accessed: February 6, 2021]

[66] Putt MS, Proskin HM. Custom tray application of peroxide gel as an adjunct to scaling and root planing in the treatment of periodontitis: Results of a randomized controlled trial after six months. The Journal of Clinical Dentistry. 2013;**24**(3):100-107. Available from: https://pubmed.ncbi.nlm.nih.gov/24660272/ [Accessed: February 6, 2021]

[67] Qing P, Huang S, Gao S, Qian L, Yu H. Effect of gamma irradiation on the wear behaviour of human tooth enamel. Scientific Reports. 2015;**5**. DOI: 10.1038/srep11568

[68] Schmeling A, Black S. An introduction to the history of age estimation in the living. In: Age Estimation in the Living: The Practitioner's Guide. 2010. pp. 1-18. DOI: 10.1002/9780470669785.ch1

[69] Bang G, Ramm E. Determination of age in humans from root dentin transparency. Acta Odontologica Scandinavica. 1970;**28**(1):3-35. DOI: 10.3109/00016357009033130

[70] Zaiontz C. Bland-Altman Plot | real statistics using excel. 2020. Available from: https://www.real-statistics.com/reliability/interrater-reliability/bland-altman-analysis/bland-altman-plot/ [Accessed: December 5, 2020]

[71] Berchtold A. Test–retest: Agreement or reliability? Methodological Innovations. 2016;**9**:205979911667287. DOI: 10.1177/2059799116672875

[72] Galton F. Finger Prints by Francis Galton [Facsimile Edition]. 64–65. 1892. Available from: http://www.safedoc.com/BiometricBits.htm

[73] Sarajlić N, Cihlarz Z, Klonowski EE, Selak I, Brkić H, Topić B. Two-criteria dental aging method applied to a Bosnian population: Comparison of formulae for each tooth group versus one formula for all teeth. Bosnian Journal of Basic Medical Sciences. 2006;**6**(3):78-83. DOI: 10.17305/bjbms.2006.3150

[74] Megyesi MS, Ubelaker DH, Sauer NJ. Test of the Lamendin aging method on two historic skeletal samples. American Journal of Physical Anthropology. 2006;**131**(3):363-367. DOI: 10.1002/ajpa.20446

[75] Jiménez NP, Santiesteban GM, Rodríguez ED, Hernández AZ. Análisis comparativo de la técnica de Lamendin y la técnica de González-Colmenares para estimación de edad en adultos. Revista Mexicana de Medicina Forense y Ciencias de la Salud. 2017;**2**(2):11-22. Available from: http://revistas.uv.mx/index.php/RevINMEFO/article/view/2724

Chapter 3

Forensic DNA Phenotyping

Murad Ali Rahat, Sumaia Saif, Muzafar Shah, Akhtar Rasool, Fazal Akbar, Shahid Ali and Muhammad Israr

Abstract

The basis for DNA analysis used in forensic research is the concept that everyone, excluding monozygotic twins, shares a genetic makeup. By directly comparing the genetic profile of short tandem repeats obtained from biological samples of unknown origin to a reference sample profile, DNA collected from biological samples can individually identify this material. The requirement for a reference sample for comparison is one of the main drawbacks of this method. Studies looking at the connection between specific polymorphisms and specific phenotypic traits are multiplying, and the results are encouraging for forensic sciences. Externally visible characteristics (EVCs), such as skin color, eye color, hair color, height, facial features, and male baldness pattern, can be inferred from biological samples for forensic purposes. This technique is called "forensic DNA phenotyping" (FDP). Therefore, without the necessity for a reference sample for comparative analysis, FDP offers additional information about the subject to which a specific biological sample belongs. So that this new technology does not encourage segregation or ethnic persecution of certain population groups, several ethical and legal considerations need to be made. Despite this, using these techniques to guide investigations and identify both suspects and victims has helped in a number of actual incidents.

Keywords: deoxyribonucleic acid, skin color, eye color, polymorphism, biological samples

1. Introduction

The basic goal of forensic DNA analysis is to create DNA profiles for identification using biological evidence. The ultimate objective is to identify the source of that biological stuff, which is the individual. Short tandem repeats (STRs), which make up most conventional DNA profiles, can fail to match suspects or entries in DNA databases when created from crime scene samples. In these situations, the donor of the crime scene sample is still unknown, and the evidence cannot be used to support the case any further. The prediction of outwardly visible characteristics (EVCs) from DNA is known as forensic DNA phenotyping [1].

Forensic DNA phenotype (FDP) looks at certain regions of the genome that are connected either directly or indirectly for normal variance in physical appearance between individuals, circumventing the limits of DNA databases and ancestry testing alone. In order to forecast head hair pigmentation, skin pigmentation, eye pigmentation, and other phenotypic features, researchers have created systems like IrisPlex and

Snipper 2.5 that leverage single nucleotide polymorphism (SNP) multiplexing [2, 3]. Additional traits may be predicted through further research.

SNPs, which are single base alterations, or INDELS, which are insertions or deletions that take place at a particular region in the genome, are used in these experiments. These variants not only provide novel leads but also enable the generation of phenotypic profiles from DNA materials as little as 60 pg./l, which is a significant reduction from the published ranges required for a conventional STR profile [3, 4].

2. Advancements in forensic DNA typing

Molecular biology techniques are always improving, opening up new ways to effectively genotype difficult forensic materials and extract genetic material. These have mainly concentrated on the study of genetic marker types that are different from those used in traditional STR typing to help identify humans [5–7]. SNP typing provides an alternate tool for investigations in circumstances where STR typing is unsuccessful. Due to the smaller amplicon size, SNPs can be useful in genotyping highly degraded DNA [8–10].

2.1 Identity informative SNPs

Comparative to conventional testing, which is still difficult, the identification of informative SNPs could be a substantial tool for the identification of individuals [11]. These SNPs will have minimal heterogeneity within particular groups but strong heterozygosity across populations. Consequently, to research the heterozygosity and heterogeneity of various human groups, population-specific informative SNPs are needed [12].

2.2 SNPs for intelligence gathering

SNPs examined for forensic purposes do not directly establish identity, but they can give information that helps detectives focus their search for a positive match. When STR profiling cannot reliably identify an individual, this is advantageous (either from no matches to a database or where no profile can be obtained from degraded remains). Due to the uniqueness of these alleles for particular groups [9, 13–16] or due to their relationship with variations in hair and eye color [2, 16], certain SNP markers found on nuclear and mitochondrial DNA have been employed in forensic investigations of genetic ancestry.

2.3 Phenotype-informative SNPs

Genes implicated in complex traits like EVCs have been identified by genome-wide association studies (GWAS) [17, 18]. The combined effects of several genes that regulate the synthesis or localization of melanin determine the human pigmentation in skin, hair, and eye color [17]. Differential skin, hair, and eye color have been found to be substantially correlated with a number of SNPs [18]. The discovery of genetic markers that infer height, hair and shaft shape [17], facial features [19], and male pattern baldness [20, 21] is a further area of potential SNP typing for externally apparent attributes.

3. DNA phenotyping

3.1 Eye color

Eye color is one the most valuable colors among the phenotypic characteristics, which ranges from dark shades to a light blue shade through intermediate (such as hazel, gray, green, and yellow) colors. These differences follow a similar pattern to the color of hair and skin due to the number of melanosomes and the amount of melanin present in the outer layer of the iris; brown eye color has high melanin amount than blue eye color [22]. This phenomenon was conformed through phenotyping tools (Irisplex) developed and validated. The Irisplex system consisted of six SNPs present among different genes (IRF4, TYR, OCA2, SLC24A4, SLC45A2, and HERC2). The accuracy (>90%), was checked both on admixed and on homogeneous population throughout the world [23–27]. Along with these results, some Asian population did not demonstrate the same results [28]. When the accuracy of intermediate eye color was matched with blue and brown, it showed very lower accuracy [4, 29, 30]. A study by Popiech et al. [31] revealed gene–gene interaction among the three primary pigment genes (OCA2, TYRP1, and HERC2) related with green eye color, despite the difficulty in predicting these intermediate colors, encouraging the development of future prediction models. Gender is another topic that has been considered in relation to the manipulation of eye pigmentation. It has been noted that men tend to have lighter eyes than women do in various European countries [25, 31, 32]. More research will be required to assess this link because no genetic element has yet been identified to account for this variation.

3.2 Hair color

One of the most noticeable EVCs with a wide range of phenotypes is hair color, along with skin and eye colors. Red/yellow pheomelanin and brown/black eumelanin are two distinct types of proteins that are primarily responsible for defending hair color [32]. People with red hair have more pheomelanin than eumelanin, whereas people with dark hair have more eumelanin than those with red hair, and people with blond hair have less of each form of melanin overall [33]. These changes in hair color increased in Europe, which changed from ancestral hair color due the human mating preferences [32]. In the process of melanogenesis control by numerous genes, MC1R was one of the first to determine a strong perceptive rule for red hair, freckles, and fair skin. Later, successive associations of other genes were also found such as HERC2, SLC24A5, and SLC45A2, and based on 22 SNP, a predictive model was developed, which showed 81–93% accuracy for each hair color category [34]. In 2013, modification was made in the Irisplex system by adding 18 hair color markers, and the name was changed to HIrisplex System. This system consisted of markers such as SLC45A2, MC1R, OCA2, HERC2, TYRP1, IRF4, TYR, ASIP, SLC24A4, and EXOC2 genes, and some genes were added from the model previously created by Branicki et al. [35]. It can reach similar accuracy values (75–92%) [36]. Despite good result of HIrisplex System, there were some difficulties in the prediction of hair color, which changes with age (mainly in childhood). Majority of the studies avoid younger population for sampling reason because they have different phenotypes in the early stage of life. So prediction model used for phenotyping showed accurate results for adult samples as compared to childhood; the markers of age-dependent phenotypes partially predict that the blond hair color and accuracy for hair color is lower (80% for black, 78% for red, and 69% for brown) through HIrisplex. In a study carried out on young population aged 6 to 13, the result explained that hair color darkening occurred at stage of life above then 13 year of age. Hirisplex incorrectly predicted blond hair color of the younger population aged 6 to 13. So additional new SNP sets are needed to overcome this error rate [3].

3.3 Skin color

One of the most diversely researched pigmentation phenotypes is skin color. The development of skin pigmentation is thought to have resulted from an evolutionary reaction to the concentration of ultraviolet light between various planet zones. Contrarily, in locations distant from the Equator, where UV light intensity is lower and lighter skin is permitted, areas adjacent to the Equator would have higher UV intensity and a higher frequency of dark hair color [37].

The evolutionary factor makes the phenotype/genotype linkage research difficult; besides, this phenomenon also creates difficulties in the correlation studies that are only applicable to a single specific population. However, the linkage found in admixed populations did not have the same bias as in more homogeneous populations, such as Europeans [38]. Beside these research studies, other studies were performed on same populations, which were not able to distinguish skin color among different groups of African, Native Americans, and Asian [39]. Based on these evolutionary differences, a skin prediction model was created consisting of 36 SNPs from 16 pigmentation genes [4]. The developed prediction model has the ability to predict skin color; colors were categories of scale, three category scale (dark, light, and dark-black) to five category scale (dark-black, pale, dark, intermediate, and very pale). The prediction accuracies for the three-category scales have 72%–97%, while that for five-category scales have 83%–97. Some of the previous studies have been found associated with admixed population for genes such as HERC2 [40], SLC24A5 [39, 41], and SLC45A2 [42, 43]. These studies can be used for future applications. HIrisplex-s, HIrisplex, and Irisplex were grouped into a single tool, which is openly available for hair, skin, and eye color prediction using genotypes date from DNA (from https://hirisplex.erasmusmc.nl/); different eye, hair, and skin colors are predicted on the basis of probability values obtained from the prediction model having 41 markers.

3.4 Height

Until 2008, various investigations were conducted and found a few genes to be associated with human height. The results of various association studies revealed that 54 loci had a direct correlation with height variance. The number of genetic markers rose over time, reaching 180 in 2010 and 700 in 2014 [40, 43–46]. The discovered genes played a major role in the growth signaling pathway as well as the expression of genes in crucial tissues including fibroblast growth factor [40]. Despite the enormous number of height-related variants, they have little scientific significance. While the initial studies obtained accuracy values of ~65%, the most current studies failed to increase this value >75%, demonstrating the large number of SNPs still to be discovered and how complex this trait may be [47]. Moreover, human height may have a different etiology other than genetic aspects, such as gestational (placental features and maternal health aspects such as nutrition, pathologies, and drugs), hormonal, and environmental factors (nutrition and lifestyle) mainly during childhood [48]. Among all EVCs, the facial shape prediction is one of the major objectives when studying phenotyping, glimpsing the final "DNA facial composite". The face morphology is studied from the distances between facial landmarks, as nostril width, lip width, distance between eyes, and face height. Some of the genetic markers associated with facial features are initially found in syndromes and facial deformity disease studies (such as cleft palate, cleft lip, and other craniofacial dysplasia). Some of these markers are then correlated to craniofacial development and consequently linked to the normal variation of facial shape [19]. For example, PAX3 gene encodes a transcription factor present in neural crest cells, which was also related to Waardenburg syndrome and was later associated with the nasion position [49]. Other candidate genes have been identified following patterns similar to PAX3, such as PRDM16 and TP63. However, similar to height determination, each of these genetic markers seems to have a small contribution toward the total face morphology [19]. The approach used by Claes et al. [50] based primarily on data obtained from admixed populations employs a first step in which the sample ancestry and gender are used to create a base face, in which data from 24 SNPs will subsequently be used, to convey nose, lips, face roundness, jaw, chin, and supraorbital crest information to this primary face. Other studies also found significant associations with facial width, eyebrow width, distance between eyes, columella inclination, nose bridge width, nostril width, and mouth shape [51, 52].

3.5 Baldness

According to research, the genetic basis of male pattern baldness, also known as androgenic alopecia, is significant and accounts for roughly 80% of its heritability. The X chromosomes q12 region, which contains the genes AR and EDA2R, which are, respectively, directly linked to the synthesis of androgen receptor and ectodysplasin A2 receptor, the 20p11 region, and the genes EBF1, TARDBP, and HDAC9, which have the potential for prediction, are among the many loci that may be implicated. These five SNPs exhibit the highest association values as yet, with a total accuracy of 76.2%. The accuracy rises to 86.4% with the inclusion of 10 markers (rs1050286, rs1160312, rs4679955, rs962458, rs6625150, rs12007229, rs913063, rs6945541, rs1041668, and rs966881), showing that when paired with stronger markers, even SNPs with low prediction accuracy can have high accuracy [20, 52, 53].

3.6 Age estimation

It has been shown that age estimation of an individual benefits from epigenetic study using DNA methylation detection methods, which take a different approach from those previously shown here (SNP typing mostly). Because it completes the data gathered by the EVCs outlined here, age estimation is essential in the forensic context. By establishing the age range of the sample source, one may reduce the number of potential suspects while simultaneously improving the final face composite [54]. DNA methylation changes during the course of an individual's life; levels increase during childhood and then decrease once they reach adulthood [55]. These changes can be detected and used to determine an individual's age from biological samples with as few as seven markers and a variety of origins (tissues and bodily fluids) and in a variety of contexts (either from human remains or from a crime scene) with high accuracy (deviation of 3.15 years relative to the real chronological age) [56].

3.7 Ancestry

Certain DNA markers can disclose an individual's ancestry, allowing for a thorough investigation of their biogeographic contributions (Africa, Europe, Asia, and Amerindian). As a result, ancestry informative markers (AIMs) can be utilized to

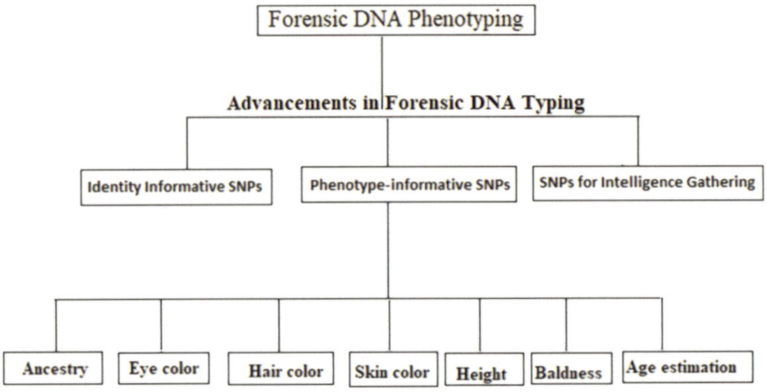

Figure 1.
Flowchart showing the search results and screening process.

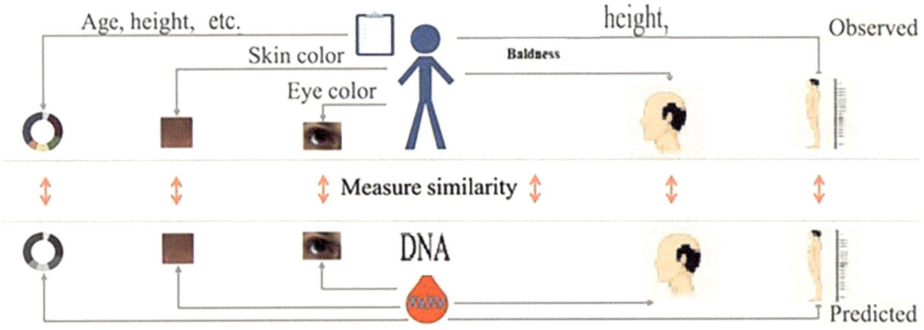

Figure 2.
Current and emerging trends in human identification.

infer someone's ancestry, providing evidence to support potential witnesses or even providing fresh information regarding forensic evidence [54]. But when evaluating someone's appearance, ancestry knowledge cannot be the only thing taken into account. One must understand the difference between ancestry and the false notion of race: a person's percentage of ancestry will not always match how they appear on the outside. When AIMs demonstrate that there is no correlation between exterior traits (ethnic background) and evolutionary biogeographic origin, this is especially clear in samples of admixed populations (**Figures 1** and **2**) [54].

4. Conclusion

A complete "DNA facial composite" is already a spectacle for forensic prediction, according to the research presented here on genetic phenotyping. A set of genetic markers were found to be used to precisely predict the majority of human extremely visible characteristics for forensic use faster than ever. To confirm data from the global population and to examine the relationship between genetic markers and ancestry or other populations, additional diverse population studies are needed. These techniques are still utilized in forensic investigations with excellent accuracy, despite some ethical and legal challenges.

Conflict of interest

The authors declare no conflict of interest.

Author details

Murad Ali Rahat[1,2], Sumaia Saif[2], Muzafar Shah[3], Akhtar Rasool[1], Fazal Akbar[1], Shahid Ali[1] and Muhammad Israr[2*]

1 Centre for Biotechnology and Microbiology, University of Swat, KP, Pakistan

2 Department of Forensic Sciences, University of Swat, KP, Pakistan

3 Centre for Animal Sciences and Fisheries, University of Swat, KP, Pakistan

*Address all correspondence to: israr@uswat.edu.pk

References

[1] Kayser M, Liu F, Janssens ACJ, Rivadeneira F, Lao O, van Duijn K, et al. Three genome-wide association studies and a linkage analysis identify HERC2 as a human iris color gene. American Journal of Human Genetics. 2008;**82**(2):411-423

[2] Hart KL, Kimura SL, Mushailov V, Budimlija ZM, Prinz M, Wurmbach E. Improved eye- and skin-color prediction based on 8 SNPs. Croatian Medical Journal. 2013;**54**(3):248-256. DOI: 10.3325/cmj.2013.54.248

[3] Walsh S, Chaitanya L, Clarisse L, Wirken L, Draus-Barini J, Kovatsi L, et al. Developmental validation of the HIrisPlex system: DNA-based eye and hair colour prediction for forensic and anthropological usage. Forensic Science International Genetics. 2014;**9**:150-161. DOI: 10.1016/j.fsigen.2013.12.006

[4] Walsh S, Liu F, Wollstein A, Kovatsi L, Ralf A, Kosiniak-Kamysz A, et al. The HIrisPlex system for simultaneous prediction of hair and eye colour from DNA. Forensic Science International Genetics. 2013;**7**(1):98-115

[5] Israr M, Shahid AA, Rahman Z, Zar MS, Shahzad MS, Husnain T, et al. Development and characterization of a new 12-plex ChrX miniSTR system. International Journal of Legal Medicine. 2014;**128**(4):595-598. DOI: 10.1007/s00414-014-1009-x

[6] Musgrave-Brown E, Ballard D, Balogh K, Bender K, Berger B, Bogus M, et al. Forensic validation of the SNPforID 52-plex assay. Forensic Science International Genetics. 2007;**1**(2):186-190. DOI: 10.1016/j.fsigen.2007.01.004

[7] Fondevila M, Phillips C, Naveran N, Fernandez L, Cerezo M, Salas A, et al. Case report: Identification of skeletal remains using short-amplicon marker analysis of severely degraded DNA extracted from a decomposed and charred femur. Forensic Science International Genetics. 2008;**2**(3):212-218. DOI: 10.1016/j.fsigen.2008.02.005

[8] Budowle B, Allard MW, Wilson MR, Chakraborty R. Forensics and mitochondrial DNA: Applications, debates, and foundations. Annual Review of Genomics and Human Genetics. 2003;**4**(1):119-141. DOI: 10.1146/annurev.genom.4.070802.110352

[9] Phillips C, Salas A, Sánchez JJ, Fondevila M, Gómez-Tato A, Álvarez-Dios J, et al. Inferring ancestral origin using a single multiplex assay of ancestry-informative marker SNPs. Forensic Science International. Genetics. 2007;**1**(3-4):273-280. DOI: 10.1016/j.fsigen.2007.06.008

[10] Zar MS, Shahid AA, Shahzad MS, Shin K-J, Lee HY, Lee S-S, et al. Forensic SNP genotyping with SN aPshot: Development of a novel In-house SBE multiplex SNP assay. Journal of Forensic Sciences. 2018;**63**(6):1824-1829

[11] Freire-Aradas A, Fondevila M, Kriegel A-K, Phillips C, Gill P, Prieto L, et al. A new SNP assay for identification of highly degraded human DNA. Forensic Science International Genetics. 2012;**6**(3):341-349. DOI: 10.1016/j.fsigen.2011.07.010

[12] Budowle B, van Daal A. Forensically relevant SNP classes. BioTechniques. 2008;**44**(5):603-610. DOI: 10.2144/000112806

[13] Butler JM. Advanced topics in forensic DNA typing: methodology.

Academic press; 2011. DOI: 10.1016/c2011-0-04189-3

[14] Kayser M, De Knijff P. Improving human forensics through advances in genetics, genomics and molecular biology. Nature Reviews Genetics. 2011;**12**(3):179-192

[15] van Oven M, Vermeulen M, Kayser M. Multiplex genotyping system for efficient inference of matrilineal genetic ancestry with continental resolution. Investigative Genetics. 2011;**2**(1):1-14. DOI: 10.1186/2041-2223-2-6

[16] Valverde L, Köhnemann S, Cardoso S, Pfeiffer H, de Pancorbo MM. Improving the analysis of Y-SNP haplogroups by a single highly informative 16 SNP multiplex PCR-minisequencing assay. Electrophoresis. 2013;**34**(4):605-612. DOI: 10.1002/elps.201200433

[17] Sulem P, Gudbjartsson DF, Stacey SN, Helgason A, Rafnar T, Jakobsdottir M, et al. Two newly identified genetic determinants of pigmentation in Europeans. Nature Genetics. 2008;**40**(7):835-837

[18] Han J, Kraft P, Nan H, Guo Q, Chen C, Qureshi A, et al. A genome-wide association study identifies novel alleles associated with hair color and skin pigmentation. PLoS Genetics. 2008;**4**(5):e1000074

[19] Liu F, Van Der Lijn F, Schurmann C, Zhu G, Chakravarty MM, Hysi PG, et al. A genome-wide association study identifies five loci influencing facial morphology in Europeans. PLoS Genetics. 2012;**8**(9):e1002932

[20] Marcińska M, Pośpiech E, Abidi S, Andersen JD, van den Berge M, Carracedo Á, et al. Evaluation of DNA variants associated with androgenetic alopecia and their potential to predict male pattern baldness. PLoS One. 2015;**10**(5):e0127852. DOI: 10.1371/journal.pone.0127852

[21] Liu F, Hamer MA, Heilmann S, Herold C, Moebus S, Hofman A, et al. Prediction of male-pattern baldness from genotypes. European Journal of Human Genetics. 2015;**24**(6):895-902. DOI: 10.1038/ejhg.2015.220

[22] Sturm R. Eye colour: Portals into pigmentation genes and ancestry. Trends in Genetics. 2004;**20**(8):327-332. DOI: 10.1016/j.tig.2004.06.010

[23] Walsh S, Liu F, Ballantyne KN, van Oven M, Lao O, Kayser M. IrisPlex: A sensitive DNA tool for accurate prediction of blue and brown eye colour in the absence of ancestry information. Forensic Science International. Genetics. 2011;**5**(3):170-180. DOI: 10.1016/j.fsigen.2010.02.004

[24] Dembinski GM, Picard CJ. Evaluation of the IrisPlex DNA-based eye color prediction assay in a United States population. Forensic Science International Genetics. 2014;**9**:111-117. DOI: 10.1016/j.fsigen.2013.12.003

[25] Kastelic V, Pośpiech E, Draus-Barini J, Branicki W, Drobnič K. Prediction of eye color in the Slovenian population using the IrisPlex SNPs. Croatian Medical Journal. 2013;**54**(4):381-386

[26] Pietroni C, Andersen JD, Johansen P, Andersen MM, Harder S, Paulsen R, et al. The effect of gender on eye colour variation in European populations and an evaluation of the IrisPlex prediction model. Forensic Science International Genetics. 2014;**11**:1-6

[27] Pośpiech E, Karłowska-Pik J, Ziemkiewicz B, Kukla M, Skowron M, Wojas-Pelc A, et al. Further evidence for population specific differences in

the effect of DNA markers and gender on eye colour prediction in forensics. International Journal of Legal Medicine. 2016;**130**(4):923-934

[28] Ruiz Y, Phillips C, Gomez-Tato A, Alvarez-Dios J, De Cal MC, Cruz R, et al. Further development of forensic eye color predictive tests. Forensic Science International Genetics. 2013;7(1):28-40

[29] Yun L, Gu Y, Rajeevan H, Kidd KK. Application of six IrisPlex SNPs and comparison of two eye color prediction systems in diverse Eurasia populations. International Journal of Legal Medicine. 2014;**128**(3):447-453

[30] Walsh S, Lindenbergh A, Zuniga SB, Sijen T, de Knijff P, Kayser M, et al. Developmental validation of the IrisPlex system: determination of blue and brown iris colour for forensic intelligence. Forensic Science International Genetics. 2011;**5**(5):464-471. DOI: 10.1016/j.fsigen.2010.09.008

[31] Pośpiech E, Draus-Barini J, Kupiec T, Wojas-Pelc A, Branicki W. Gene–gene interactions contribute to eye colour variation in humans. Journal of Human Genetics. 2011;**56**(6):447-455

[32] Sulem P, Gudbjartsson DF, Stacey SN, Helgason A, Rafnar T, Magnusson KP, et al. Genetic determinants of hair, eye and skin pigmentation in Europeans. Nature Genetics. 2007;**39**(12):1443

[33] Rees JL. Genetics of hair and skin color. Annual Review of Genetics. 2003;**37**(1):67-90

[34] Gerstenblith MR, Goldstein AM, Fargnoli MC, Peris K, Landi MT. Comprehensive evaluation of allele frequency differences ofMC1Rvariants across populations. Human Mutation. 2007;**28**(5):495-505. DOI: 10.1002/humu.20476

[35] Branicki W, Liu F, van Duijn K, Draus-Barini J, Pośpiech E, Walsh S, et al. Model-based prediction of human hair color using DNA variants. Human Genetics. 2011;**129**(4):443-454

[36] Frost P. European hair and eye color: A case of frequency-dependent sexual selection? Evolution and Human Behavior. 2006;**27**(2):85-103

[37] Jablonski NG, Chaplin G. The colours of humanity: The evolution of pigmentation in the human lineage. Philosophical Transactions of the Royal Society B. 2017;**372**(1724):20160349. DOI: 10.1098/rstb.2016.0349

[38] Maroñas O, Phillips C, Söchtig J, Gomez-Tato A, Cruz R, Alvarez-Dios J, et al. Development of a forensic skin colour predictive test. Forensic Science International. Genetics. 2014;**13**:34-44. DOI: 10.1016/j.fsigen.2014.06.017

[39] Liu F, Visser M, Duffy DL, Hysi PG, Jacobs LC, Lao O, et al. Genetics of skin color variation in Europeans: Genome-wide association studies with functional follow-up. Human Genetics. 2015;**134**(8):823-835. DOI: 10.1007/s00439-015-1559-0

[40] Weedon MN, Lango H, Lindgren CM, Wallace C, Evans DM, Mangino M, et al. Genome-wide association analysis identifies 20 loci that influence adult height. Nature Genetics. 2008;**40**(5):575-583. DOI: 10.1038/ng.121

[41] de Araújo LF, de Toledo GF, Fridman C. SLC24A5 and ASIP as phenotypic predictors in Brazilian population for forensic purposes. Legal Medicine. 2015;**17**(4):261-266. DOI: 10.1016/j.legalmed.2015.03.001

[42] Correction: Implications of the admixture process in skin color molecular assessment. PLoS One.

2014;**9**(9):e109451. DOI: 10.1371/journal.pone.0109451

[43] de A Fracasso NC, de Andrade ES, CEV W, CCF A, Zanão LR, da Silva MS, et al. Haplotypes from the SLC45A2 gene are associated with the presence of freckles and eye, hair and skin pigmentation in Brazil. Legal Medicine. 2017;**25**:43-51. DOI: 10.1016/j.legalmed.2016.12.013

[44] Allen HL, Estrada K, Lettre G, Berndt SI, Weedon MN, Rivadeneira F, et al. Hundreds of variants clustered in genomic loci and biological pathways affect human height. Nature. 2010;**467**(7317):832-838

[45] Gudbjartsson DF, Walters GB, Thorleifsson G, Stefansson H, Halldorsson BV, Zusmanovich P, et al. Many sequence variants affecting diversity of adult human height. Nature Genetics. 2008;**40**(5):609-615. DOI: 10.1038/ng.122

[46] Lettre G, Jackson AU, Gieger C, Schumacher FR, Berndt SI, Sanna S, et al. Identification of ten loci associated with height highlights new biological pathways in human growth. Nature Genetics. 2008;**40**(5):584-591. DOI: 10.1038/ng.125

[47] Guo MH, Hirschhorn JN, Dauber A. Insights and implications of genome-wide association studies of height. The Journal of Clinical Endocrinology and Metabolism. 2018;**103**(9):3155-3168. DOI: 10.1210/jc.2018-01126

[48] Liu F, Hendriks AEJ, Ralf A, Boot AM, Benyi E, Sävendahl L, et al. Common DNA variants predict tall stature in Europeans. Human Genetics. 2013;**133**(5):587-597. DOI: 10.1007/s00439-013-1394-0

[49] Paternoster L, Zhurov AI, Toma AM, Kemp JP, St Pourcain B, Timpson NJ, et al. Genome-wide association study of three-dimensional facial morphology identifies a variant in PAX3 associated with nasion position. American Journal of Human Genetics. 2012;**90**(3):478-485. DOI: 10.1016/j.ajhg.2011.12.021

[50] Claes P, Hill H, Shriver MD. Toward DNA-based facial composites: Preliminary results and validation. Forensic Science International. Genetics. 2014;**13**:208-216. DOI: 10.1016/j.fsigen.2014.08.008

[51] Fagertun J, Wolffhechel K, Pers TH, Nielsen HB, Gudbjartsson D, Stefansson H, et al. Predicting facial characteristics from complex polygenic variations. Forensic Science International Genetics. 2015;**19**:263-268. DOI: 10.1016/j.fsigen.2015.08.004

[52] Adhikari K, Fuentes-Guajardo M, Quinto-Sánchez M, Mendoza-Revilla J, Camilo Chacón-Duque J, Acuña-Alonzo V, et al. A genome-wide association scan implicates DCHS2, RUNX2, GLI3, PAX1 and EDAR in human facial variation. Nature Communications. 2016;7(1):1-11. DOI: 10.1038/ncomms11616

[53] Heath AC, Nyholt DR, Gillespie NA, Martin NG. Genetic basis of male pattern baldness. The Journal of Investigative Dermatology. 2003;**121**(6):1561-1564. DOI: 10.1111/j.1523-1747.2003.12615.x

[54] Vidaki A, Kayser M. Recent progress, methods and perspectives in forensic epigenetics. Forensic Science International Genetics. 2018;**37**:180-195. DOI: 10.1016/j.fsigen.2018.08.008

[55] Jones MJ, Goodman SJ, Kobor MS. DNAmethylation and healthy human aging. Aging Cell. 2015;**14**(6):924-932. DOI: 10.1111/acel.12349

[56] Hong SR, Jung S-E, Lee EH, Shin K-J, Yang WI, Lee HY. DNA methylation-based age prediction from saliva: High age predictability by combination of 7 CpG markers. Forensic Science International Genetics. 2017;**29**:118-125. DOI: 10.1016/j.fsigen.2017.04.006

Chapter 4

Developing a Universal Identification Model: Integrating AI and IoT Tools with DNAFIDs to Recognize COVID-19 Patients

Yogesh Pal, Vullikanti Vivek Kumar, Deepak Garg and Neeraj Kumar Verma

Abstract

DNA fingerprinting identification systems based on artificial intelligence infuse almost every facet of life. Its impact on various aspects of human health can be seen today. It has also found its importance in the identification of global COVID-19 infections, whether suspected or proven, in patients. Because of the IoT and the application of sophisticated filtering techniques to big data, it's conceivable. The technology of DNA profiling, which creates detailed profiles of individual characteristics, is a necessity. This can be incredibly helpful in the acquisition process in certain circumstances when paired with other data. Many candidates' medical and physiological factors are included in the Human Clinical Profile (HCP), as are social profile-related services. The government spends significant tax dollars vetting the physical and medical characteristics of various candidates for clinical care and purposes related to public health response. We propose a technique that may help analyze the physical traits of candidates preemptively and conduct forensic investigation for human identification, which may help reduce the cost of check-ups and other medical processes. This technique combines DNA profiling with artificial intelligence tools to pre-screen candidates for COVID-19 patients who require physical and remote monitoring. Further experiments done in a targeted manner are justification for the hypothesis.

Keywords: DNAFIDs, IoT, AI, COVID-19, HCP

1. Introduction

Compared to entirely distinct virus outbreaks or the vast majority of diverse ancient tragedies, pandemics like COVID-19 are current issues of a completely different sort. These diseases wreak havoc on communities around the world that lack immunity to them as a result, and their spread may be far faster and frequently more deadly than that of any comparable condition outbreak. It is imperative for our country to create a human database based on the medical and DNA fingerprinting ID models, which helps multi-purpose as per the requirements. India's Aadhaar Card-Unique

Identification Authority of India is required to create a twelve-digit unique number for each resident of the country in order to continuously provide benefits to hundreds of people through the use of various government insurance policies like Direct Benefit Transfer, Aadhaar with Aarogya Setu App-Enabled Biometric Group Action, and Registration Tool Methodology to be used through Central Authority Agencies. According to the following figure, discussions around Aadhaar have been contentious for a some now and are likely to continue for some time. This chapter's goal is not to get involved in that debate, but rather to highlight the urgent need for emergency protection in social programmes against "Aadhaar-related problems." Numerous such annoyances exist, frequently causing millions of people inconvenience or worse, especially those from underprivileged communities. A number of them have been listed in a number of surveys, papers, articles, statements, audits, petitions, tweets, and videos, but the warnings have largely gone unheeded. Even fervent Aadhaar proponents should give these concerns more attention (**Figure 1**).

In this chapter, we will pay particular attention to and harness India's identification models, such as the Aadhar Card, Voter ID, Passport, etc., and surpass their limitations by synchronizing IoT for practical uses through DNAFIDs in order to stop the spread of COVID19 [1, 2]. AI technology that can recognize polymers can be used to identify patients as being ill.

Many international locations perform rhetorical DNA-databases to know proprietors of crime associated stains [3]. Victimization compound to hint persons administrative body unit of measurement suspected of committing a criminal offense has been a basic boost in policing. Once compound identification is used accurately, it'll assist to convict humans administrative body have dedicated serious

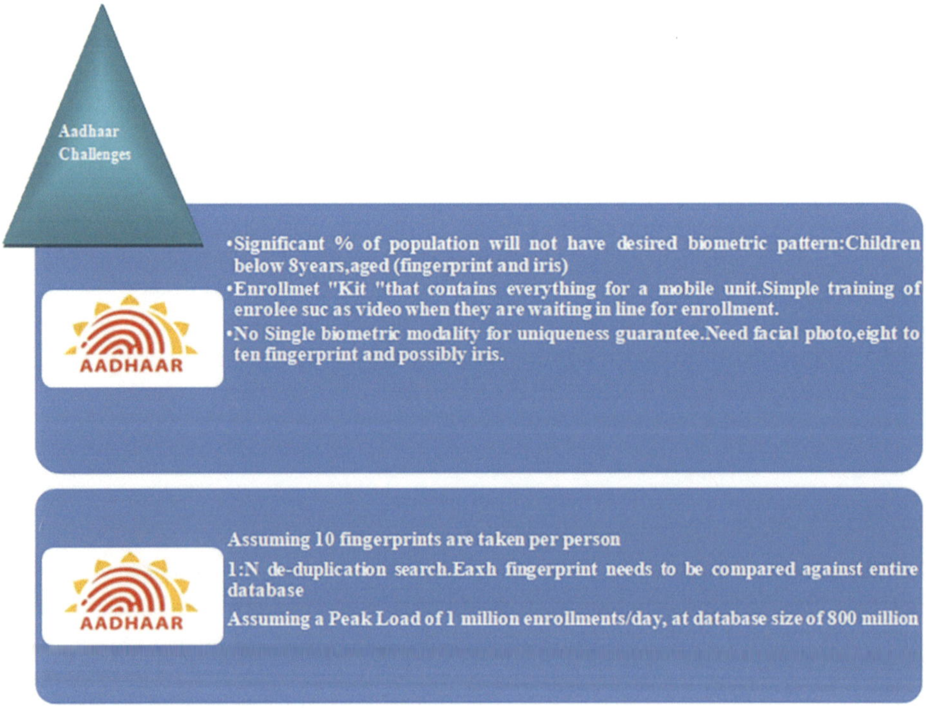

Figure 1.
Aadhaar challenges.

crimes or discharge person's administrative body unit of measurement harmless [4]. Compound data is also a pc data containing data of compound profiles. Generally there unit of measurement two distinctive sources of these compound profiles: crime scene compound samples and individuals' compound samples. The employment of compound databases in crook investigations desires associate individual's identification to be discovered completely if there's a healthy between their compound profile and a criminal offense scene compound profile. The rhetorical compound data also can assist crook investigators to line up hyperlinks between a singular suspect of a selected crime and fully completely different unresolved crimes, or can grant assist to become tuned in to plausible suspects whereas clearing fully completely different suspects inside the first degrees of associate Investigation [5]. The political and economic investments inside the implementation of rhetorical deoxyribonucleic acid databases and so the moral troubles associated to their use and growth justify inquiries into their overall performance and ancient utility. The primary characteristic of the rhetorical deoxyribonucleic acid data is to provide fits between persons, crime scene stains, that desires a delicate, enter of character profiles, and crime scene stains [5]. Our ride through these two instances indicates that rhetorical deoxyribonucleic acid statistics base accustomed be integral to become tuned in to the killers. There's associate degree current would like for higher public and coverage dialog as deoxyribonucleic acid databases amplify round the world. Some safeguards unit of measurement disbursed at the country wide or regional level, however there is associate degree absence of international requirements and a desire for larger social engagement and dialog [2]. Extensive data and deoxyribonucleic acid identification of criminals and assortment them will assist to pace up crime detection [6]. Larger deoxyribonucleic acid databases decrease crime rates, within the main in classes the place rhetorical proof is probable to be collected at the scene—e.g., murder, rape, assault, and automobile law-breaking. The prospect of beautiful a suspect in new crimes falls as databases grow, all told chance attributable to resolution effects. Back-of-the-envelope estimates of the marginal worth of stopping every crime endorse that deoxyribonucleic acid databases unit of measurement tons additional worth effective than altogether completely different frequent regulation group action instrumentality [5]. Forensic deoxyribonucleic acid databases have the manageable to forestall and see crime The introduction and growth of rhetorical deoxyribonucleic acid databases would possibly contain plausible threats to the protection of a vary of human rights. At the identical time, such databases have social edges. Supported statistics accumulated via associate degree on-line kind utilized to 628 humans in land, this paper targets to analysis the citizens' temperament to relinquish voluntarily a pattern for identification and inclusion inside the National rhetorical deoxyribonucleic acid data and so the views underpinning such a decision. Nearly one-quarter of the respondents would signify 'no', and this terrible response improved appreciably with age and education. The dominant temperament to be the inclusion of the person or girl genetic profile suggests associate degree acknowledgement of the inquiring realizable of rhetorical deoxyribonucleic acid applied sciences and a relegation of civil liberties and human rights to the background, as a result of the perceived blessings of defensive each society and so the character from crime. This reason is typically expressed by methodology of the thought that everybody residents have to be compelled to be compelled to form a contribution to the growth of the National rhetorical deoxyribonucleic acid data for motives that change from the larger define assumption that donating a pattern for identification would be useful in struggle crime to the larger concrete recommendation that everybody folks (criminals and non-criminals) have to be compelled to be compelled to be inside the data. The issues with the risks of exceptive the donation of a pattern for procedure and inclusion inside the National rhetorical deoxyribonucleic acid data unit of measurement further generally than not associated to lack of manage and inadequate or unsure pointers with reference to safeguarding individuals' facts and oversight the get right of entry to and makes use of genetic info. By activity associate degree empirically-grounded grasp of the attitudes involving temperament to relinquish voluntary a pattern for identification and inclusion throughout a National rhetorical deoxyribonucleic acid data, this resolve on the point of boot considers the citizens' perceived blessings and dangers of operative rhetorical deoxyribonucleic acid databases. These collective views is also useful for the formation of worldwide frequent moral requirements for the advance and governance of deoxyribonucleic acid databases throughout a framework throughout that the citizens' views unit of measurement taken into thought. DNA data coverage needs to search out a smart stability between these two positions, based entirely on the arrival of {a moral an moral} and ethical spectrum involving each consultants inside the neighborhood of forensics and regulation group action [7] and so the general public [8], especially, social businesses that unit of measurement a great deal of less concerned in biology [9]. DNA data for all residents than authorities concerned inside the fitness zone and in neighborhood and broad protection and regulation group action ([10], p. 601); older and immature contributors (more than sixty five or between fifteen and twenty four years, respectively) area unit these administrative body most often united with the transferring of records from deoxyribonucleic acid profile databases to native and State Security Agencies ([11], p. 143); and cognizance of the employment of deoxyribonucleic acid identification inside the identification of people accelerated markedly with employment.

In the case of Covid-19, AI functions just like the employment of facial cognizance to tune humans not sporting masks publically, or AI-based fever detection systems, as nicely as a result of the method of statistics gathered on digital systems and cell networks to music people's latest movements, have contributed to the lawgiver group action of restraining measures inside the course of the confinement aimed toward containing the happening, for one durations. Chinese net search Brobdingnagian Baidu has developed a tool the utilization of infrared and facial cognizance technological ability that scans and takes footage of larger than 2 hundred humans per minute at the Qinghai train depot in capital of Red China. In Moscow, authorities unit of measurement the usage of automatic facial cognizance technological ability to scan investigation digital footage in academic degree try and choose out current arrivals from China, positioned at lower place quarantine for worry of Covid-19 infection. The assessment resolve regarding explored this digital or IoT-based applied sciences that unit of measurement obtaining used for containment of pandemic unfold of COVID-19 round the globe. IoT intervention to fight the pandemic unfolds of COVID-19 and to grant fitness offerings at some purpose of this vulnerable quantity. AI (AI) is collaborating in several roles to limit the human interaction and involvement to battle con to the COVID-19 pandemic. Services like disorder investigation, early warnings and alerts, digital tending facilitate, prognosis and prognosis, facts verification over social media, dominant social distancing and activity the lockdown, remedy and cures, method and inspecting COVID-19 take a look at samples, investigation and observation folks even once a personal is carrying a face-mask and so the likes unit of measurement obtained from the AI-based technologies. Native use of IVR as if Aaroyga Setu in land has been in addition placed tremendous for tending facilitate, coverage and knowledge series on COVID-19.

1.1 However computing will assist combat COVID-19

Artificial brain is contributory to combat the COVID-19 pandemic. Comes associated to material medical, scientific and consultation room care, or quality analysis to attenuate contagion has determined an essential ally in statistics science to make development and supply results. The pandemic brought on through COVID-19 is that the initial world public fitness disaster of the twenty 1st century. And today, a number of AI-powered initiatives based entirely on records science, computer learning or 'big data', area unit being used across an enormous vary of fields to predict, offer associate degree proof for and management the one among a kind eventualities caused by suggests that of the fitness crisis. As regards coding system of AI to analysis, work appears to be progressing at a modest pace.

2. DNAFIDs (DNA fingerprinting identification system) database: functions and uses

In 1989, the first instance of a parentage dispute resolved by victimization in India used compound procedure technology. Since then, compound science has been employed to establish person identity, from crook instances to natural rhetorical identification, as well as to decrease the incidence of paternity and maternity disputes [12].

The innovative development in forensic science of DNA fingerprinting aids in identifying people and is a crucial tool for molecular research that promotes human breeding. By analyzing distinctive DNA patterns, the DNA fingerprinting model was essential in identifying specific persons among millions of others. A technique called DNA fingerprinting finds several minisatellites in a genome at once to create a pattern that is specific to a certain person. In this research project, we analyzed DNA fingerprinting-based identification and developed a DNA fingerprinting-based identification model together with a DNA database management system for 360-degree interlinking, meaning that all services and advancement will be advanced by DNAFIDs and database.

Y. Pal, S. Kumar, M. Singh et al. [2] To improve all administrations and innovations, for instance, DNAFIDs and data sets will be utilized. The UML class model approval process through FSM has been addressed by Yogesh Pal [1]. This is demonstrated by a production of the progress table examined for Interlinking of DNA Models with Aadhaar Real-Time Records for Enhanced Authentication.

3. IoT and AI-based smart healthcare: applications

DNA Profiling, artificial intelligence (AI), and the internet of things (IoT) are interconnected research areas that have a significant influence on the creation of improved personalized healthcare systems. Research into smart healthcare is extensive [12], there is a vast body of literature in the field of smart health care that covers IoT, IoMT, medical signals, AI, edge, and cloud computing at varying rates and utilizing various methodologies. To the best of our knowledge, there has not been a comprehensive review of contemporary edge and cloud computing, IoT, IoMT, medical signal utilization and fusion, privacy, and security in the field of smart health care. The goal of this survey was to provide a formal classification, a detailed comparative context, and privacy and security in smart health care for IoT, IoMT, edge and cloud computing. The study examined the utilization of IoT, IoMT, and medical signals as well as the combination of sensors, edge computing [13]. The use of artificial intelligence (AI) technologies in the medical industry has a long history of advancement. Diverse research teams have also been motivated to keep investigating AI in-depth as a result of several persistent issues and obstacles in the medical industry. AI technology has become increasingly frequently used in the medical industry as a result of the development of cutting-edge technologies like the Internet of Things (IoT), cloud computing, big data, and 5G mobile networks. Additionally, the comprehensive integration of AI and IoT technology enables the steady enhancement of medical diagnosis and treatment capacities in order to deliver services to the public more successfully.

4. Proposed model: Integrating AI and IoT tools with DNAFIDS to recognize COVID-19 patients

An RDBMS was used to build the DNA fingerprinting database system. Based on the current widely used open source programme SQL Server, the database is implemented. Entity relationship model is shown in **Figure 2**. (ERD). First, we determined the 10 entities and 4 relationships that Chen's ERD notation used to express the ERD. Using the ERD as a foundation, a table-like model is built. In **Figure 2**, the "PCR" and "CE" entities are divided into two tables, respectively: "PCR" and "PCR well" and "CE" and "CE well". The wells in the plate are described and precisely located using these tables, which also provide extra information. The source of the sample connects all the parties, and they are all linked together by fundamental details like primers, panels, and detection tools.

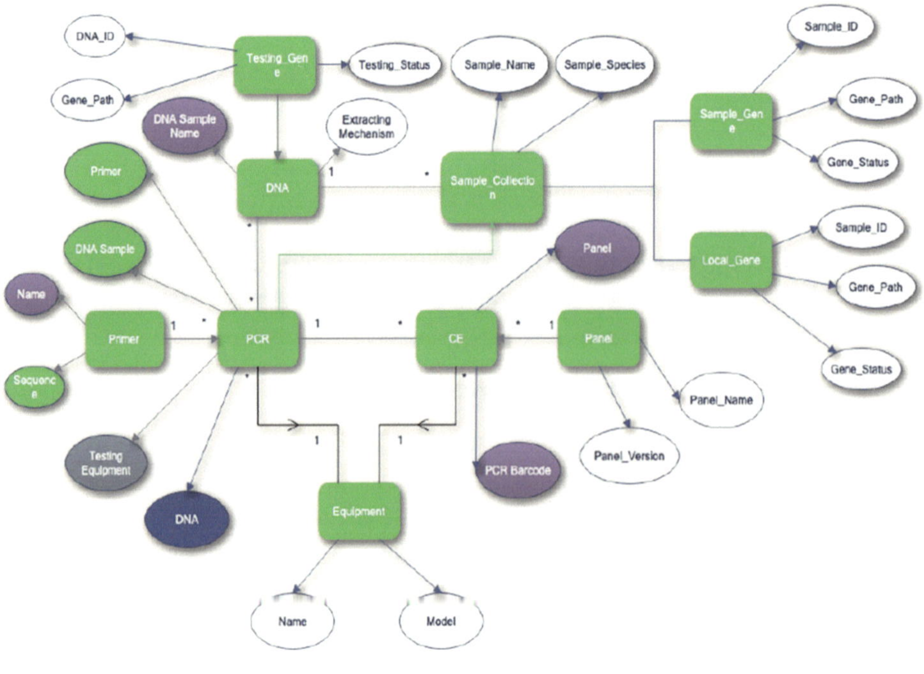

Figure 2.
E-R diagram for DNA fingerprinting database system.

Basic data, testing data, and fingerprint data are all included in the DNA fingerprint database. Bar code numbers or IDs are used to link these databases together. The DNA Fingerprinting Database System holds fingerprint data and fingerprint picture information in separate files in order to address the issue of fingerprint data compatibility with various human primers. The fingerprint data file is linked to the fingerprint image's storage path information, and after that, the fingerprint data file path information is saved in the fingerprint data's basic information table. The fingerprint data file only has to be updated with new data when loading and updating fingerprint data and fingerprint images. The issue of slow operations, such as those caused by queries that access a database, is avoided by this method. With the use of the Adhaar Card database, DFD of AI & IoT, DNAFIDs, and other technical support, we examine the theoretical foundations of the suggested model (**Figure 3**).

From the aforementioned DFD and ER diagram, it can be inferred that DFD is an effective modeling technique for a variety of research topics, allowing one to show both the static and dynamic behavior of the system. The work mentioned above is based on the validation method used by DFD for Integrating AI and IoT Tools with DNAFIDS to Recognize COVID-19 Patients. Additionally, this DFD created a DNAFIDs model that illustrates the entire process of DNA profiling [2]. A variety of test cases taken from the FSM are used to validate the proposed model for DNA profiling/DNAFIDs.

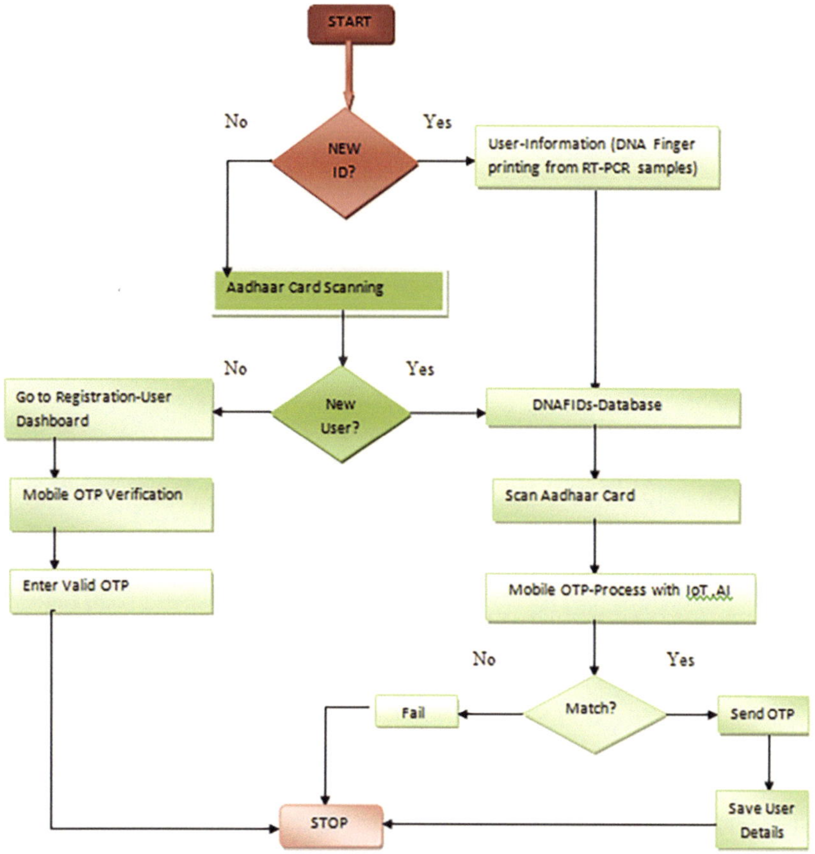

Figure 3.
DFD: Integrating AI and IoT tools with DNAFIDS to recognize COVID-19 patients.

5. Conclusion

The modular architecture efficiently demonstrated the benefits of combining AI and IoT tools with DNAFIDS to identify COVID-19 patients. DNA biometrics for more uniqueness in USID to add an additional layer of security With the aid of API, contemporary security technologies, and internet accessibility, the integrated technique aids in communicating a state of concern to the government. There will be no need to use several IDs.

Conflict of interest

All authors declared that they do not have any conflict of interest.

Author details

Yogesh Pal[1*], Vullikanti Vivek Kumar[2], Deepak Garg[3] and Neeraj Kumar Verma[4]

1 Post-Doctoral Fellow, School of Computer Science Engineering and Technology, Bennett University, Uttar Pradesh, India

2 Research Fellow, Department of Electrical and Computer Engineering, College of Design and Engineering, National University of Singapore, Singapore

3 School of Computer Science Engineering and Technology, International Affairs and Corporate Outreach, Bennett University, Uttar Pradesh, India

4 Department of ICAITECH, The ICFAI University, Jaipur, India

*Address all correspondence to: er.yogeshpal15@gmail.com

References

[1] Singh YP, Kumar S, Singh M. Analysis and designing a dna fingerprinting based identifications (dnafids) model and database management system. Reliability: Theory & Applications. 2021;**16**(1):152-160. DOI: 10.24412/1932-2321-2021-161-152-160

[2] Pal Y, Kumar S, Singh M, Dwivedi S. Validation of DNAFIDs model through finite state machine. Reliability: Theory & Applications. 2021;**16**(3):160-167. DOI: 10.24412/1932-2321-2021-363-160-167

[3] van der Beek K. Measuring The Effectiveness and Efficiency of Forensic DNA databases. 26 International Symposium on Human Identification. 2016

[4] DNA Databases and Human Rights|Forensic Genetics Policy Initiative. http://www.dnapolicyinitiative.org/resources/dna-databases-and-human-rights/

[5] Santos F, Machado H, Silva S. Forensic DNA databases in European countries: Is size linked to performance? Life Sci. Soc. Policy. 2013;**9**:12

[6] Panneerchelvam S, Norazmi MN. Forensic DNA profiling and database, Malays. Journal of Medicine Science. 2003;**10**:20-26

[7] Amorim A. Opening the DNA black box: Demythologizing forensic genetics. New Genetics and Society. 2012;**31**(3):259-270

[8] Williams R, Johnson P. Inclusiveness, effectiveness and intrusiveness: Issues in the developing uses of DNA profiling in support of criminal investigations. The Journal of Law, Medicine & Ethics. 2005;**33**(3):545-558

[9] Wilson-Kovacs D, Wyatt D, Hauskeller C. 'A Faustian bargain?' Public voices on forensic DNA technologies and the national DNA database. New Genetics and Society. 2012;**31**(3):285-298

[10] Gamero JJ, Romero JL, Peralta JL, Carvalho M, Corte-Real F. Spanish public awareness regarding DNA profile databases in forensic genetics: What type of DNA profiles should be included? Journal of Medical Ethics. 2007;**33**(10):598-604

[11] Gamero JJ, Romero JL, Peralta JL, Corte-Real F, Guille'n M, Anjos MJ. A study of Spanish attitudes regarding the custody and use of forensic DNA databases. Forensic Science International. 2008;**2**(2):138-149

[12] Alshehri F, Muhammad G. A comprehensive survey of the internet of things (IoT) and AI-based smart healthcare. IEEE Access. 2021;**9**:3660-3678. DOI: 10.1109/ACCESS.2020.3047960

[13] Xia Lu Z et al. Application of AI and IoT in clinical medicine: Summary and challenges. Current Medical Science. 2021;**41**(6):1134-1150. DOI: 10.1007/s11596-021-2486-z

Chapter 5

Comparison of Risk Factors and Preventable Causes of Unnatural Deaths from 1990 to 2017

Nimra Ishfaq

Abstract

The aim of this study is to identify the possible risk factors and preventable causes of unnatural deaths. By doing so recommendations can be made to authorities to help create a safer environment for society. A retrospective, descriptive study was carried out and randomized samples were collected. A total of 772 medico-legal autopsy reports from 1990 to 2017 were divided into two groups for analysis and data collection. Group A consists of autopsy reports from 2016 to 2014 and Group B consists of autopsy reports from 1990 to 1996. Information such as age, sex, occupation, and brief facts about the case were collected. Nature of violence and cause of death were also studied. The trends between the two groups were then noted and compared and discussed. The commonest cause of death is homicidal in nature. The second highest nature of violence is accidental cases for example falling from trees, roofs, or brawling or falling due to old age. Firearms are the most commonly used weapons. The most likely to be at risk of unnatural death is a young, healthy male adult of age group of 21–30 and 31–40. Females of age group of 21–30 and 11–20 are more at risk.

Keywords: risk factors, preventable causes, unnatural deaths, firearms, sharp-edged weapons

1. Introduction

Over the past few decades, there has been a noticeable rise in crime and a corresponding rise in cases of unnatural deaths. In a study carried out in Karachi in 2009, out of 2090 medico-legal autopsies 98.7% were found to be unnatural deaths [1]. A death is considered unnatural if it is homicidal, suicidal, accidental, or due to some other violent or unexplained cause [2]. It is in the best interest of society to work toward reducing the number of medico-legal deaths. This will lessen not only the economic burden but also the psychological and emotional stress that results in depression and post-traumatic stress disorder [3]. Such circumstances reduce the overall productivity and mental health of a society. It is necessary to reduce deaths. A risk factor is anything that increases the likelihood to suffer harm. It may be sex, occupation, or even geographical location.

In a study for risk factors of unnatural deaths, fatal accidental intoxication was found to be associated with male gender, use of heroin, and use of cannabis. Death from intoxication/injury of undetermined intent was associated with heroin use as well as binge drinking of alcohol and previous psychiatric hospitalization. Death from suicide was associated with previous suicide attempts and sedative use [4].

The aim of this study is to identify possible risk factors and preventable causes of unnatural deaths. By doing so recommendations can be made to authorities to help create a safer environment for society.

2. Materials and methods

- Study type: A retrospective, descriptive study

- Sampling technique: Randomized samples were collected. A total of 772 medico-legal autopsy reports from 1990 to 2017 were divided into two groups for analysis and data collection. Group A consists of autopsy reports from 2016 to 2014 and Group B consists of autopsy reports from 1990 to 1996.

- Information like age, sex, occupation, and brief facts about the case was collected. Nature of violence and cause of death were also studied. The trends between the two groups were then noted and compared and discussed.

- Place of study: Conducted in Forensic Medicine department KEMU, Lahore, Pakistan.

- Duration of study: 5 months from March to June (2017)

- Inclusion and exclusion criteria: Severely decomposed bodies and cases where cause of death was unidentified were excluded

3. Results

Table 1 illustrates the age wise distribution that shows that most likely healthy young male adults are at risk to suffer death. For analysis, the data has been divided into two groups. Group A comprises of 665 cases from the year 2014–2016 and Group B comprises of 107 cases from 1990 to 1996. Group A shows that the highest number of unnatural deaths for males was in 2014 (210, 91.7%). However, the highest number of deaths for females was in 2016 (44, 18.6%). The ratio of male to female deaths is the same for Group B (4.35:1) and for the year 2016 in Group A highlighted in yellow in **Table 1**. It is interesting to note that two samples of data almost 20 years apart have presented with the same ratio and could provide basis for further study. The age group most likely to be affected for males is 21–30 with 2014 presenting with the most cases (57) followed by 2015 (43), 2016 (41), and group B (34). The second highest affected age group is 31–40. The most cases are presented in 2014 (51) followed by age group 41–50.

Group A							Group B	
	2016 (236)		2015 (200)		2014 (229)		1990–1996 (107)	
Range (years)	*Female*	*Male*	*Female*	*Male*	*Female*	*Male*	*Female*	*Male*
0–10	8	3	4	5	2	8	3	2
11–20	7	14	9	11	4	12	5	12
21–30	11	41	16	43	7	57	5	34
31–40	5	43	5	39	3	51	2	14
41–50	6	37	2	37	1	34	3	12
51–60	5	32	1	17	0	28	2	10
61–70	2	22	0	9	1	19	0	3
>70	0	0	1	1	1	1	0	0
Total	**44** (18.6%)	**192** (81.3%)	**38** (19.0%)	**162** (81.0%)	**19** (8.3%)	**210** (91.7%)	**20** (18.6%)	**87** (81.3%)

Table 1.
Age-wise distribution.

The trend seems to be similar for both Group A and B for males but the trend is different for females. For females, the age group most likely affected is also 21–30 but this time the highest number of cases is seen to be in 2015 (16) followed by 2016 (11), 2014 (7), and group B (5). It is followed by 11–20 as the second highest affected age group with 2015 of group A again presenting the most number of cases (9).

Table 2 illustrates the nature of violence in which homicide is the commonest for both sexes. The year with the highest number of cases for males is 2014 (92) followed by 2016 (88) and Group B (82). 2015 has the lowest number of cases (77) for males. Females present with the highest cases in 2016 (31) followed by 2015 (27), 2014 (18), and group B with 16 cases.

Group A							Group B	
	2016 (236)		2015 (200)		2014 (229)		1990–1996 (107)	
Type	*Female*	*Male*	*Female*	*Male*	*Female*	*Male*	*Female*	*Male*
Homicide	17	53	19	61	15	79	9	59
Suicide	0	0	0	0	0	0	0	0
Accidental	1	14	1	4	0	5	0	13
RTA	0	12	3	0	0	1	2	9
Industrial	0	0	0	0	0	0	0	1
Burn	6	6	1	4	0	0	5	0
Strangulation	7	3	3	8	3	7	0	0
Total	**31**	**88**	**27**	**77**	**18**	**92**	**16**	**82**

Table 2.
Nature of violence.

Line chart 1.

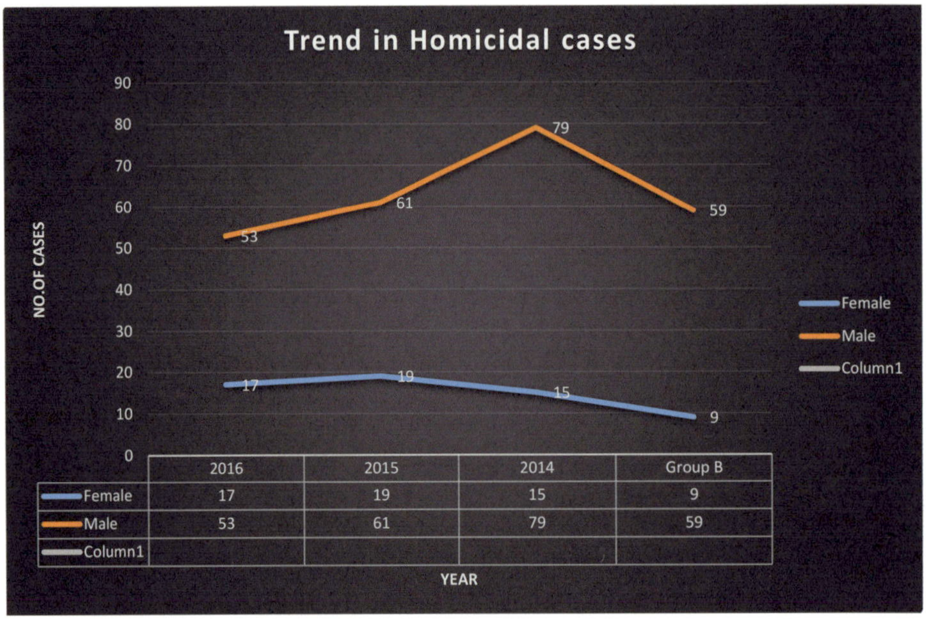

The highest number of homicidal cases is 79 in 2014 for males and 19 cases in 2015 for females. The lowest number of homicidal cases is 53 in 2016 for males and 9 cases in group B for females. The second highest nature of violence is accidental cases for example falling from trees and roofs or brawling or falling due to old age. The highest number of cases was present in 2016 (14) followed by group B (13) for males. RTA (road traffic accidents) is third commonest with the highest number in 2016 (12) followed by group B (9) for males. The trend seems similar to that seen in accidental cases. Strangulation is the fourth commonest with the highest number of cases being 8 in 2015 for males and 7 in 2016 for females. The trend for burn cases is erratic. Both males and females presented with equal number of cases (6) in 2016 but in 2015 the ratio for males to females is 4:1 and in Group B only 5 female burn cases were found. 2014 presented zero burn cases. Number of cases due to industrial causes and suicide was almost zero.

Table 3 illustrates the commonest mechanism of death is hemorrhagic vascular with the most number of cases being 75 for males in 2014 followed by Group B (69). For females, the highest is 16 in 2016 followed by 14 in 2015. However, there is only 1 case of hemorrhage in 2014 for females. The second most common mechanism is neurogenic/shock/coma. Both 2016 and group B have the highest cases for males (15). For females, the highest number of cases is 10 in 2015. Septicemia/infection is highly uncommon in Group A but is prominent with 10 cases for males in Group B. Asphyxia is more common in females in 2016 (7 cases) but more common in males in 2015 (8) and 2014 (7). In Group B, there are zero cases of deaths by asphyxia.

Table 4 shows that firearms are the most commonly used weapons in 2014 (54 cases) and Group B (53 cases) followed by 29 cases in 2015 and 28 cases in 2016. The highest number of cases with blunt weapon/means used are in 2015 (46 cases) and 2014 (44). Compared to the other choice of weapons, sharp edge weapons are uncommon with the highest number of cases being only 17 in Group B and the lowest number of cases being 6 in 2014.

DOI: http://dx.doi.org/10.5772/intechopen.109032

Group A							Group B	
	2016 (236)		2015 (200)		2014 (229)		1990–1996 (107)	
Type	*Female*	*Male*	*Female*	*Male*	*Female*	*Male*	*Female*	*Male*
Hemorrhagic/ Vascular	16	48	14	52	1	75	2	69
Neurogenic/ Shock/coma	0	15	10	9	2	9	8	15
Septicemia/ Infection	1	1	0	2	0	0	3	10
Asphyxia	7	3	3	8	3	7	0	0
Total	24	67	27	71	6	84	13	94

Table 3.
Mechanism of death.

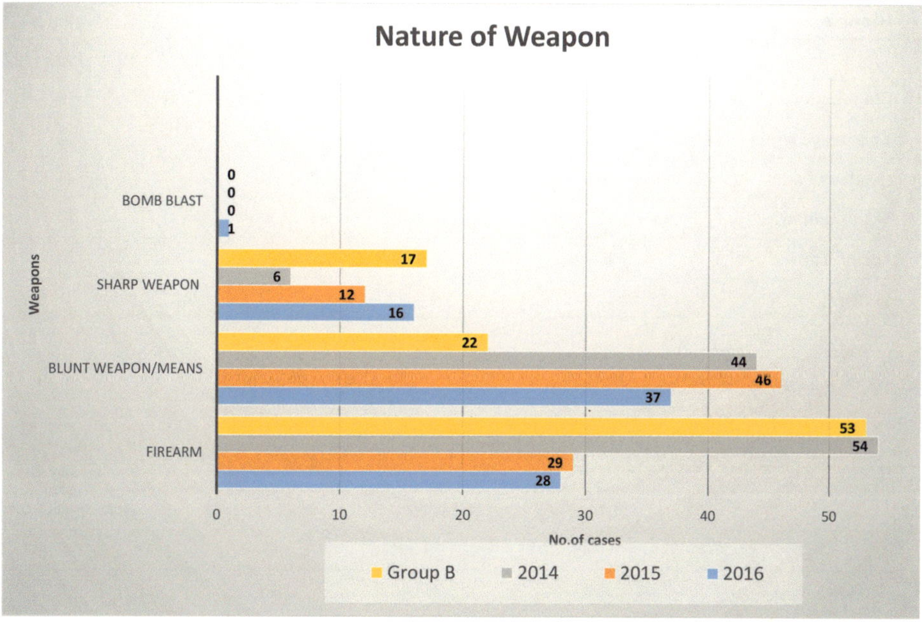

Table 4.
Nature of weapon.

In **Table 5** in Group A, the organ with the highest rate of damage is the brain. 2015 presents with the highest number of cases 48 followed closely by 2014 with 47 cases and 2016 with 39 cases. But Group B has only 17 cases that involve the brain, while the organ most damaged is the lung with 40 cases followed by 2014 (30 cases), 2015 (16), and 2016 (18). For liver highest number of cases is 24 in Group B and 13 in Group A (2014). The second highest organ damaged in Group B is heart with 26 cases but the cases decrease in number in Group A with the highest number of cases being only 14 in 2014. Most number of cases involving intestines in Group B is 18. The number of cases involving kidneys decrease from Group B (10) to Group A (2016 with 4 cases).

Group A				Group B
	2016 (236)	2015 (200)	2014 (229)	1990–1996 (107)
Brain	39	48	47	17
Heart	8	5	14	26
Lungs	18	16	30	40
Liver	9	5	13	24
Diaphragm	1	3	6	12
Stomach	7	3	8	21
Intestines	12	4	12	18
Kidney	4	5	2	10

Table 5.
Organs and viscera involved.

Group A				Group B
	2016 (236)	2015 (200)	2014 (229)	1990–1996 (107)
Chest injury	17	9	11	10
Abdominal injury	11	10	15	20
Head injury	30	22	20	13
Multiple injuries	12	8	10	10
Bony fractures	10	6	8	20
Limbs	2	4	2	0

Table 6.
Associated injuries.

Group A				Group B
	2016 (236)	2015 (200)	2014 (229)	1990–1996 (107)
T. B	45	29	35	4
COPD	22	23	30	0
CILD(lung)	35	34	35	3
CILD (liver)	12	8	14	0
Meningitis/ encephalitis / coronary disease	3	2	5	0

Table 7.
Natural deaths.

Table 6 illustrates that deaths involving head injury alone are the highest in group A with 30 cases in 2016 followed by 2015 (22) and 2014 (20). In Group B deaths involving abdominal injury and bony fractures are more common with 20 cases each.

Table 7 highlights that tuberculosis has been a major cause of death in 2016 with 45 cases and in 2014 with 33 cases. Chronic inflammatory lung disease is the second commonest cause with 35 cases in 2016 (**Table 8**).

Group A				Group B	
Geographical Locations	**2016 (236)**	**2015 (200)**	**2014 (229)**	**1990–1996 (107)**	**Total**
City Division	131	90	115	42	378
Civil Lines Division	52	35	44	23	155
Cantonment Division	33	30	29	15	107
Iqbal Town Division	10	24	15	14	68
Model Town Division	8	10	11	11	40
Sadar Division	10	11	15	2	38
Total	234	200	229	107	772

Table 8.
Geographical locations.

4. Discussion

The most likely to suffer from an unnatural death is a healthy young male adult. The age group with the most frequent deaths is 21–30 for both sexes with the second highest age group being 31–40 for males and 11–20 for females. For the highest age group, 21–30 for males, 2014 presented with the most cases (57) followed by 2015 (43), 2016 (41), and group B (1990–1996) showed 34 cases.

A study carried out in Peshawar, Pakistan studied a total of 3265 autopsies. 2839 were male and 426 were female showing a ratio of 6.66:1 [5]. In a study carried out in India in 2020, 10.3% of total deaths were unnatural and were greater in the population aged 10 to 45 years. The unnatural mortality rate was found to be 0.84 per 1000 among the male population and 0.49 per 1000 among the female population [6]. However, in another study in India in 2014, 74% of the victims of unnatural deaths were found to be adolescents and were 3 times more common than other age groups [7]. In a study in Shanghai, China in 2015, the male-to-female ratio of unnatural deaths was 2.02:1, and the average age was 40.9 [8]. These findings may probably reflect the more active role males have in society. Young men are more prone to imitate violent acts displayed on entertainment media or peer pressure to participate in criminal activities [9].

The commonest nature of violence as shown in **Table 2** is homicide followed by strangulation, burn, accidental, and then RTA (road traffic accident) in Group A. The trend is similar in Group B, however, there are zero strangulation cases and accidental cases are the second commonest. The trend in homicidal cases as seen in **Table 2** indicates that homicidal cases involving females are much less in number than males. This is similar to several other studies in Pakistan indicating that this may be significant [10–12]. The slope rises from right to left, which shows that female homicidal cases have increased in the last 30 years but it is the opposite case for males. In addition, there is a sharp increase in male homicidal cases in 2014 (79 cases).

A study conducted in South Africa noted the frequency of death from homicide and factors associated with homicide death. The study took place between 2000 and 2008 and reported 536 homicide-related deaths. The overall homicide rate was 66 deaths per 100, 000 person-years of observation [13]. A study in the Netherlands among 2130 homeless persons found the most frequent cause of death to be unnatural deaths (26%). Of these suicide and homicide were responsible for 50% [14]. Another study in Ontario, Canada investigated homicide cases over a period of 1999 to 2012 and found that victims were mostly young males of 15–29 years. The trend of homicides followed an upward increase and the overall rate was found to be 3.85 per 100,000 population [15].

A study by Kleeman and Fischer in 1994 examined a group of homicide victims over the years 1978–1988 to determine the causes of their injuries. Out of 251 cases, they found that 51.4% of homicide victims had injuries due to blunt trauma, 31.9% were due to sharp trauma and 29.5% were from strangulation. Shootings were found to be less common (18.7%) and other types of traumas were around 4.0%. The most common victims of blunt force trauma and sharp trauma were male, 51.9% and 33.6%, respectively. Females demonstrated injuries due to blunt trauma (50.8%) as well as strangulation (47.5%). Women were commonly murdered by the aggressor's bare hands within the setting of conflicts in relationships. In 36.7% of all cases, injuries were caused by a combination of aggressive traumas [16].

In yet another study from Western Norway, cases of 196 homicide victims from 1985 to 2009 were investigated. The median age of the victims was 35 years, including both genders. 113 of the victims were male and 83 were female. Most of the victims were killed by blunt trauma, sharp injury, or gunshot wound. The body region most often injured was found to be the head area. Female victims were more likely to be killed by strangulation than male victims [17].

An analysis of female homicide victims during a 10-year period was carried out in Taiwan. Among 220 adult victims, 114 were killed by intimate partners and 106 were killed by non-intimate partner offenders. The most common site of injuries was the neck and the upper limbs, respectively. The most common causes of death were strangulation and sharp force injury. The area of heart was injured more frequently in victims attacked by intimate partners than by other types of offenders [18].

The male-to-female ratio for burn cases in 2016 is 1:1 but in Group B, the only burn cases were of 5 females. This may be due to the honor killings that are now less common because of a more educated society. Burn victims accounted for 10.79% of medico-legal deaths studied in Kanpur, India over a period of 1 year [19]. In a study in Cairo, Egypt over a five-year period (2006–2010), around 3981 cases of autopsies were investigated. Out of these cases, 106 (2.66%) were found to be burn victims [20].

A total of 109 cases of death due to fatal burns were studied in Mumbai, India from 2014 to 2015. Cases were studied with respect to marital status, alleged history of dowry death, manner of death, history of psychiatric illness, chronic diseases, previous suicidal attempts, etc. Out of the 109 cases, females accounted for 92 cases (84.4%). Accidental deaths were 71 in number (65.14%). Sixty-seven cases (61.47%) of death due to septicemia and 42 (38.53%) died due to shock [18].

In yet another study in Nagpur, India, 384 cases of medicolegal deaths were studied. It was found that deaths due to burning accounted for 21.6% of all cases. Female victims were seen more than males (74.2%) with a male–female ratio equal to 1:2.9. Most of the victims of burn deaths were between 11 and 40 years with peak at 21–30 years (47.1%). The commonest manner of death by burning was accidental in nature (75%) by suicidal and homicidal burning [21].

Table 3 illustrates that the most common mechanism of death is hemorrhagic/ vascular followed by neurogenic shock/coma and then asphyxia while septicemia is the least common in both groups. The results of **Tables 2** and **3** can be explained after looking at **Table 4**, which presents the choice of weapon. Firearm is the most frequently used weapon in both group B and 2016 of group A, whereas blunt weapon/means is the more common choice of weapon in 2015 and 2014 of group A. This reflects that ownership of firearms in society is not kept under proper supervision and may be in the hands of unlicensed owners. Theft and robberies are carried out more and more with firearms

[22]. In 2016, 251,000 people died from firearm injuries around the world [23]. Blunt weapons and means are now more common than they were 30 years ago in group B. This may be due to the increase in violence and crime rates and gangs. In 2020, around 1,313,105 violent crimes were reported in the United States, which was an increase from the year 2019 when 1,250,393 violent crimes were reported [24].

Table 5 reveals that in the last 30 years, the most likely damaged organ has changed from lungs to the brain. Also, cases involving the heart, liver, stomach, intestines, and diaphragm have decreased but cases involving kidneys have increased in number. **Table 6** of associated injuries helps to shed light on the findings of **Table 5**. These cases are where the major injury related to death is abdominal injury alone or head injury alone or chest injury alone. The cases of head injuries (20 cases) in group B have shown an increase of almost 50% that is up to 72 cases in Group A. Abdominal injuries on the other hand occurred more frequently in group B. Cases involving chest injuries are second most frequently occurring.

There is plenty of data in similar studies carried out in Pakistan that corresponds to our findings that head injuries are most common in homicidal cases followed by Chest injuries. A study carried out in Karachi in 2012 found that head injuries were at 44.2% and the second commonest were chest injuries at 28.5% [25]. In Brazil from 2015 to 2018, head injuries were identified in 168 homicide victims and accounted for 68.3%. The study also found an association between the presence of head injuries and number of injuries ($p < 0.05$) [26].

Table 7 titled natural deaths showcases interesting results. Out of 772 medico-legal autopsies, there were 113 cases (14.6%) of tuberculosis [TB] and 75(9.7%) cases of chronic inflammatory lung disease [CILD]. This displays that TB and other respiratory diseases are risk factors. The incidence of increase in Tb may be largely due to the rise in population that the economy cannot support resulting in cramped living spaces. In 2019, approximately 1.21 million HIV-negative patients died of TB [27]. According to World Health Organization (WHO), the association between TB and poverty is mediated by overcrowding, poorly ventilated housing, malnutrition, smoking, stress, social deprivation, and poor social capital [28]. For effective control of spread of TB, there is need for development of an effective surveillance system, improved speed of diagnoses of cases, improved healthcare in rural areas, and increased provision of healthcare staff and laboratory facilities [29].

According to data collected in the United States in 2020, the top 3 causes of preventable deaths were poisoning, motor vehicles, and falls accounting for 86% of all preventable causes [30]. According to a study carried out in Finland, accidental deaths and suicide mortality rates of men were 2–13 and 2–3 times those of women, respectively. Deaths due to homicide were less prevalent among either sex [31]. In 2010, a study in Germany reported a total of 14,441 unnatural deaths (suicide, traffic accidents, and homicide). Of those, 10,021 subjects (69.4%) committed suicide, 3942 (27.3%) died in traffic accidents, and 478 (3.3%) were murdered. Suicide death rates were 3 times higher in men than women [32]. A Suicide appears to be a risk factor for unnatural deaths and may be prevented by awareness of mental health issues. Seminars may be held on mental health awareness and pamphlets can be published with information on recognizing suicidal tendencies in people prone to anxiety and depression. A study in the United Kingdom investigated the prevalence of suicide ideation in patients with psoriasis. Patients with psoriasis were found to have an increased risk of depression, anxiety, and suicidality. The study took place from 1987 to 2002 and estimated 10, 400 diagnoses of depression, 7100 diagnoses of anxiety, and 350 diagnoses of suicidality and were attributable to psoriasis annually [33].

Study of risk factors and preventable causes of unnatural death allows for making of health policies, which may help to prevent rise in cases of unnatural deaths. A death is considered unnatural if it is homicidal, suicidal, accidental, or due to some other violent or unexplained cause. The preventable causes include homicide, suicide, accidents, etc. Homicide death is death at the hands of one human being to another human being. Accidental deaths are described as deaths occurred due to accidents. Suicide is death voluntarily or intentionally by a human being to his or herself. Some unnatural deaths may have an undetermined cause that cannot be found by autopsy [34]. A study conducted in Germany aimed to identify frequency and causes of unnatural deaths among infants, 339 cases were investigated over a three-year period (from 1998 to 2001). The frequency of unnatural deaths was found to be 5.0% (n = 17). The causes of death included head injury (n = 7), where n = number of cases, suffocation (n = 5), poisoning (n = 2), neglect (n = 2), and septicemia due to aspiration of a foreign body (n = 1) [35].

Homicide, Suicide, and accidental deaths or undetermined causes of unnatural deaths may decrease the mental health of a society. A study carried out in Denmark, in 2001 by Hiroeh and Appleby, showed that 25% of 17,892 psychiatric patients died from unnatural causes. Patients with schizophrenia or other diagnosed mental disorders were shown to be at increased risk for death by homicide. Alcoholics and drug users were at increase for death by both homicide and accidents, and risk of death by suicide was highest among drug users [36].

Suggestions can be made to health policymakers to decrease such causes. Homicide can be prevented by improved law enforcement and surveillance of areas where homicide deaths are more likely to occur. In a study, in 2018 in United States, data on 54,170 deaths was collected and 24% were found to be due to homicide. Increased security around areas where homicidal deaths are more likely to occur will help to decrease the frequency of homicidal deaths [37].

According to a study carried out in the United States by Post and Mason in 2021, surveillance on gun usage and gun policy may decrease homicide due to firearms. The results of the study showed that the Federal Assault Weapons Ban (FAWB) (1994–2004) had a positive impact in discouraging firearms. The FAWB prevented 11 public mass shootings during the decade it was in effect. Linear regression analysis of the data showed that continued implementation of the FAWB would have prevented 30 public shootings and saved the lives of 339 people and 1139 injured people [38].

Deaths from unnatural causes are preventable. Identifying risk factors may allow health policymakers a greater depth of understanding of the needs of the population when designing public health guidelines. Appropriate safety measures can be put into effect more easily. Previous literature on the subject is sparse. The aim of this study is to address this gap and identify the risk factors associated with unnatural deaths in a third-world country. In this study, factors such as male gender, younger age, and geographical areas with higher crime rates have been identified to increase the likelihood of unnatural death. In a study by Wilson and Gaugrhan in 2019, factors associated with unnatural mortality in patients with serious mental disorders were studied. Patients with serious mental disorders who died from unnatural causes were likely to be of younger age, male or have a psychiatric diagnosis, or have been recently discharged from a psychiatric hospital [39].

The importance of reducing deaths related to unnatural causes is many folds. Firstly, the economic burden on society can be reduced and psychological stress of families suffering from loss of loved ones can be reduced. Such emotional distress leads to mental distress furthering the risk of mental health disorders. The overall productivity of society can be reduced if these stressors remain prevalent. A study analyzing pattern of deaths in Dhaka Medical College, India found 1725 unnatural deaths out of 1772 total deaths. The frequency of causes was 69% road traffic accidents, 12% homicide, 8% suicide, and 3% natural. Burn, electrocution, and others causes comprised the rest [40].

Identifying factors and their reduction can help to increase the socioeconomic wealth and leads to improved well-being of a society. A healthy society can lead to improvement in functioning and can lead to further success such as in economy and infrastructure. A study in Lucknow India from 2008 to 2012 identified the causes and epidemiological aspects of unnatural deaths in the elderly. There were 3165 male victims and 1240 female victims. Unnatural deaths were higher in rural (64%) than in urban (37%) areas. Accidental deaths were the most common manner of unnatural deaths (59%), followed by suicidal deaths (34%) and homicidal deaths (7%) [41]. Rural areas where socioeconomic wealth is low show higher risk of unnatural deaths indicating that improvement in socioeconomic wealth of society will improve well-being and will likely decrease the risk of unnatural deaths.

This present study aims to fill the gap in current research on preventable causes of unnatural deaths and their associated risk factors. Further research on this topic can benefit society by helping to further supplement understanding of the areas that need improvement and can, therefore, decrease the likelihood of unnatural deaths.

5. Conclusion

The most likely to be at risk of unnatural death is a young, healthy male adult of age group of 21–30 and 31–40. Females of age group of 21–30 and 11–20 are more at risk. The most common nature of violence is homicide followed by strangulation, burn, accidental, and then RTA (road traffic accident). The commonest mechanism of death is hemorrhagic/vascular followed by neurogenic shock/coma and then asphyxia while septicemia is the least common. Firearm is the most frequently used weapon followed by blunt means/weapon and Sharp-edge weapon. Frequently associated injury is head injury followed by chest injury. TB, CILD, and other respiratory diseases are likely to be preventable causes.

Author details

Nimra Ishfaq
Independent researcher, Lahore, Pakistan

*Address all correspondence to: nimraishfaq209@gmail.com

References

[1] Farhat HM, Hassan Q, Naz R. Spectrum of medico-legal deaths in metropolis of Karachi: An autopsy based study. Pakistan Journal of Medicine and Dentistry. 2013;**1**:1.012-1.011. n. pag. Print

[2] Kitulwatte IDG, Edirisinghe PAS, PratheepaMendis HKNL, Wijesinghe PR, Fernando A, Abeyrathne AARM. Study on the pattern of unnatural deaths of women brought for medico-legal autopsy. Sri Lanka Journal of Forensic Medicine, Science & Law. 2017;**8**(1): 13-22. DOI: 10.4038/sljfmsl.v8i1.7789

[3] Keyes KM, Pratt C, Galea S, et al. The burden of loss: Unexpected death of a loved one and psychiatric disorders across the life course in a national study. The American Journal of Psychiatry. Aug 2014;**171**(8):864-871. DOI: 10.1176/appi.ajp.2014.13081132. PMID: 24832609; PMCID: PMC4119479

[4] Olsson MO et al. Risk factors for unnatural death: Fatal accidental intoxication, undetermined intent and suicide: Register follow-up in a criminal justice population with substance use problems. Drug and Alcohol Dependence. 2016;**162**:176-181. DOI: 10.1016/j.drugalcdep.2016.03.009 Accessed 18 Dec. 2019

[5] Hussain KZ, Naeem M, Adil M. Analysis of autopsy record of unnatural deaths in Peshawar district. Journal of Postgraduate Medical Institute. Web. 2013;**27**(4):392-396

[6] Panda BK, Mishra US. Unnatural death in India. Journal of Biosocial Science. May 2021;**53**(3):367-378. DOI: 10.1017/S0021932020000231. Epub 2020 May 13. PMID: 32398177

[7] Debata PK et al. Causes of unnatural deaths among children and adolescents in Northern India – A qualitative analysis of postmortem data. Journal of Forensic and Legal Medicine. 2014;**26**:53-55. DOI: 10.1016/j.jflm.2014.06.001. Accessed 18 Nov. 2021

[8] He M et al. Unnatural deaths in Shanghai from 2000 to 2009: A retrospective study of forensic autopsy cases at the shanghai public security bureau. PLoS One. 2015;**10**(6):e0131309. DOI: 10.1371/journal.pone.0131309. Accessed 30 Jan. 2022

[9] Office of the Surgeon General (US). Chapter 4 – Risk factors for youth violence. Youth Violence: A Report of the Surgeon General. U.S. National Library of Medicine, 01 Jan. 1970. Web. 10 July 2017

[10] Marri MZ, Bashir MZ. An epidemiology of homicidal deaths due to rifled firearms in Peshawar Pakistan. Journal of College of Physicians and Surgeons Pakistan. Web. 2010;**20**(2):87-89

[11] Bashir MZ, Saeed A, Khan D, Aslam M, Iqbal J, Ahmed M. Pattern of homicidal deaths in Faisalabad. Journal of Ayub Medical College, Abbottabad. 2004;**16**(2):57-59

[12] Mustafa YG, Memon MU. Spectrum of unnatural deaths in Hyderabad: An autopsy based study. Journal of Dow University of Health Sciences. Web. 2010;**6**:381-382

[13] Otieno G, Marinda E, Bärnighausen T, Tanser F. High rates of homicide in a rural South African population (2000-2008): Findings from a population-based cohort study. Population Health Metrics. 2015;**13**:20. DOI: 10.1186/s12963-015-0054-0. PMID: 26300697; PMCID: PMC4545817

[14] Slockers MT, et al. [Homeless adults' most frequent cause of death is suicide or murder]. Nederlands Tijdschrift voor Geneeskunde. 2018;**162**:D2626. Available from: pubmed.ncbi.nlm.nih.gov/29543143/

[15] Lachaud J, Donnelly PD, Henry D, Kornas K, Calzavara A, Bornbaum C, et al. A population-based study of homicide deaths in Ontario, Canada using linked death records. Int J Equity Health [Internet]. [cited 2022 Dec 8]. 2017;**16**(1):133. Available from: https://pubmed.ncbi.nlm.nih.gov/28738872/

[16] Fischer J et al. Types of trauma in cases of homicide. Forensic Science International. 1994;**68**(3):161-167. DOI: 10.1016/0379-0738(94)90355-7 Accessed 4 Mar. 2020

[17] Kristoffersen S et al. Homicides in Western Norway, 1985-2009, time trends, age and gender differences. Forensic Science International. **238**(2014):1-8. DOI: 10.1016/j.forsciint.2014.02.013. Accessed 26 Sept. 2021

[18] Fong W-L et al. Adult femicide victims in forensic autopsy in Taiwan: A 10-year retrospective study. Forensic Science International;**266**(2016):80-85. DOI: 10.1016/j.forsciint.2016.05.008 Accessed 2 Feb. 2022

[19] Gupta RK, Srivastava AK. Study of fatal burns cases in Kanpur (India). Forensic Science International. 1988;**37**(2):81-89. DOI: 10.1016/0379-0738(88)90096-5 Accessed 12 May 2021

[20] Afify MM et al. Fatal burn injuries: A five year retrospective autopsy study in Cairo City, Egypt. Egyptian Journal of Forensic Sciences. 2012;**2**(4):117-122. DOI: 10.1016/j.ejfs.2012.08.002 Accessed 8 Feb. 2022

[21] Namdeorao AV, Godbole HV. Study of burn deaths in Nagpur, Central India. Burns. 2006;**32**(7):902-908. DOI: 10.1016/j.burns.2006.03.001 Accessed 30 Dec. 2020

[22] Duggans M. More guns, more crime. Journal of Political Economy. n.d. n. pag. Print

[23] More than 250,000 People Worldwide Died from Gun Injuries in 2016: Report. AP NEWS. 29 Aug. 2018. Available from: apnews.com/article/4e1e8cd0436f7c07d9525a16716b01f5. Accessed 12 Oct. 2022

[24] U.S.: Reported Violent Crime 2018. Stat. Available from: www.statista.com/statistics/191129/reported-violent-crime-in-the-us-since-1990/

[25] Farhat MC, Khan AW, Malik L, Malik M, Parveen K. An autopsy based study of pattern of firearm. Volume 3 • Issue 6 • 1000165 Emergency Med ISSN: 2165-7548 EGM, an open access journal Mirza et al., Emergency medicine. 2013;**3**:6 DOI: 10.4172/2165-7548.1000165

[26] Cavalcanti AL et al. Head and face injuries in brazilian homicide victims – A retrospective study. Annals of Maxillofacial Surgery. 2021;**11**(1):103. DOI: 10.4103/ams.ams_158_20 Accessed 13 Mar. 2022

[27] Deaths from TB - 2018 Deaths. TBFacts. 31 Aug. 2020. Available from: tbfacts.org/deaths-from-tb/

[28] Tuberculosis Control in Vulnerable Groups. WHO. World Health Organization; n.d., Web. 12 July 2017

[29] Zaman K. Tuberculosis: A global health problem. Journal of Health, Population, and Nutrition. 2010;**28**(2): 111-113. Available from: www.ncbi.nlm.nih.gov/pmc/articles/PMC2980871/. DOI: 10.3329/jhpn.v28i2.4879

[30] Available from: https://injuryfacts.nsc.org/all-injuries/deaths-by-demographics/top-10-preventable-injuries/data-details/

[31] Junno J-A et al. Unnatural-cause mortality patterns of Northern Finnish men and women diverge in adolescence – A 52-year follow-up. Preventive Medicine Reports. 2021;**22**:101337. DOI: 10.1016/j.pmedr.2021.101337 Accessed 28 May 2022

[32] Lukaschek K et al. Suicide mortality in comparison to traffic accidents and homicides as causes of unnatural death. An analysis of 14,441 cases in Germany in the year 2010. International Journal of Environmental Research and Public Health. 2012;**9**(3):924-931. Available from: www.ncbi.nlm.nih.gov/pmc/articles/PMC3367287/. DOI: 10.3390/ijerph9030924 Accessed 26 Apr. 2022

[33] Kurd SK et al. The risk of depression, anxiety and suicidality in patients with psoriasis: A population-based cohort study. Archives of Dermatology. 2010;**146**(8):891-895. Available from: www.ncbi.nlm.nih.gov/pmc/articles/PMC2928071/. DOI: 10.1001/archdermatol.2010.186 Accessed 4 Nov. 2020

[34] Marri Z, Zainab S. Study on unnatural death in Mardan, Pakistan. Journal of Mohammed Medical College. Nov 2020-April 2021;**11**(2):124-125

[35] Bajanowski T et al. Unnatural causes of sudden unexpected deaths initially thought to be sudden infant death syndrome. International Journal of Legal Medicine. 2005;**119**(4):213-216. DOI: 10.1007/s00414-005-0538-8 Accessed 14 Dec. 2020

[36] Hiroeh U et al. Death by homicide, suicide, and other unnatural causes in people with mental illness: A population-based study. The Lancet. 2001;**358**(9299):2110-2112. DOI: 10.1016/s0140-6736(01)07216-6

[37] Sheats KJ et al. Surveillance for Violent Deaths — National violent death reporting system, 39 States, the District of Columbia, and Puerto Rico, 2018. MMWR. Surveillance Summaries. 2022;**71**(3):1-44. DOI: 10.15585/mmwr.ss7103a1 Accessed 15 Apr. 2022

[38] Post L, et al. Impact of firearm surveillance on gun control policy: Regression discontinuity analysis. JMIR Public Health and Surveillance. 2021;7(4):e26042. Available from: publichealth.jmir.org/2021/4/e26042/. DOI: 10.2196/26042

[39] Wilson R et al. Place of death and other factors associated with unnatural mortality in patients with serious mental disorders: Population-based retrospective cohort study. BJPsych Open. 2019;**5**(2). DOI: 10.1192/bjo.2019.5 Accessed 2 Oct 2021

[40] Rahim M, Das TC. Mortuary profile for unnatural deaths at forensic medicine department of Dhaka Medical College. Bangladesh Medical Journal [Internet]. [cited 2022 Dec 8]. 1970;**38**(2):44-47. Available from: https://www.semanticscholar.org/paper/ea87410c69ca554cb18cae20fb9df122e6621d0

[41] Kumar S, Verma AK. A study of elderly unnatural deaths in medico-legal autopsies at Lucknow locality. Medicine, Science, and the Law. 2014;**54**(3):127-131. Available from: pubmed.ncbi.nlm.nih.gov/24166690/. DOI: 10.1177/0025802413502783. Accessed 12 Oct. 2022

Chapter 6

Perspective Chapter: Sexual Cybercrime – The Transition from the Virtual Aggression to the Physical Aggression

Mohammed Hedidi

Abstract

Cybercrime is all criminal offenses committed on telecommunications networks in general and more particularly on the Internet. Sexual cybercrime promotes the transition from virtual sexual assault to physical or bodily assault, the victims of which are often women and children through intimidation and harassment as well as the absence of consent. The damage caused by the cybersex crime of the victims can lead to serious repercussions on their physical and mental health. The obligation of the fight against this social scourge has imposed its analysis on several ways to generate the means of protection because it is the only way to preserve our families and our children particularly from being victims of sexual cybercrime.

Keywords: cybercrime, sexual cybercrime, virtual aggression, physical aggression, women, children

1. Introduction

Cybercrime is a polymorphic concept that can concern classic offenses committed through digital technologies, as well as new offenses, born from the very essence of computing. it concerns all the criminal offenses committed on telecommunications networks in general and more particularly on the Internet, such a space known by the importance of the use of social networks by Internet users whose object is to carry out communications, share information, and develop private and professional relationships.

Several types of cybercrime have been counted and promote the transition from virtual sexual assault to physical or bodily assault, the victims of which are often women. In addition, the child, in the absence of consent, can be a target of cyber predators or even an object of sexual abuse and pornographic exploitation.

The psychological damage caused by psychotrauma due to sexual cybercrime isolated or associated with physical bodily aggression can manifest itself in serious psychological or even psychiatric disorders on the health of the victims.

The obligation to fight against this social scourge has imposed its analysis in order to seek means of prevention and protection of victims through the development of cyber security and the creation of legislative texts devoted to the protection of sexual cybercrime.

2. The concept of cybercrime

2.1 The cyberspace

Cyberspace is a domain where data is stored, changed, and exchanged via physical infrastructures connected to networks and systems and the electromagnetic and electronic spectrum. The Internet is a vast, unending area known as cyberspace. You can think of computer transactions as taking place in space, especially when they happen between various computers. Cyberspace is where text and images on the Internet exist. The phrase serves as a moniker for the made-up space in which a virtual object lives when used in connection with virtual reality. A building is considered to be in cyberspace if a computer generates a picture of it that enables the architect to virtually "walk in" and assess the nature of a design. An organized criminal attack on cyberspace and cyber security is known as cybercrime. Cybercrime, such as hacking into computers, can be committed through a network system, clicking on strange links, connecting to unauthorized WiFi, downloading software and files from dubious websites, consuming energy, emitting electromagnetic radiation, and other methods [1].

The National Security Presidential Directive (NSPD), published on January 9, 2008, Cyberspace is described as "the interdependent network of information technology infrastructures, including the Internet, telecommunications networks, computer systems, and embedded processors and controllers in critical industries" in the National Security Presidential Directive (NSPD), which was released on January 9, 2008. However, there is not a single definition of cyberspace in place right now. Cyberspace can be viewed as both a collection of all information systems and as the information environment in which people live in the information age. It is therefore preferable to think of cyberspace as both an information space and a network space. The first conception emphasizes the fundamental quality of information, while the second emphasizes the crucial component of network-based interconnectedness [2].

2.2 The cybercrime

The word "cybercriminal" sounds like it should be used to describe a character from a William Gibson novel, but these individuals are all too real and regularly cause havoc in our increasingly online society. In order to combat the growing use of the Internet for criminal activity, the government announced a £25 million program in April 2001 that included the establishment of a National High-Tech Crime Unit. With 43% of the population labeling cybercrime as a "concern," the internet world is becoming more open to criminal activities [3].

At an organizational level, there are differences globally in cybercrime definitions. Additionally, some organizations do not even define cybercrime. For instance, there is no official definition of cybercrime provided by the U.S. government, making it impossible to distinguish it from other common criminal offenses or other types of cyberthreats [4].

For the council of Europe cybercrime convention, cybercrime is defined as action directed against the confidentiality, integrity and availability of computer systems, networks and computer data as well as the misuse of such systems, networks, and data by providing for the criminalization of such conduct [5].

Cybercrime is a term used to describe criminal activity in which computers or computer networks are utilized as a tool and in the commission of the crime. The prevalence of online crime has increased as the PC has become essential to business, government, and entertainment. The three main components of computer crime are unauthorized access to computer systems, information alteration, and theft of protected intellectual property. Cybercrime encompasses a wide range of profit-driven criminal activity, including identity theft, email and internet fraud, efforts to steal financial accounts, and data theft from businesses. Cybercriminals employ a variety of methods to carry out cyberattacks and are constantly looking for new methods and talents to master without being concerned about being detained or arrested. Malware infection of systems and networks is a technique used to harm installed software or data. Cybercriminals also try to target websites in an effort to alter or remove information, gain unauthorized access to, or modify databases. Cybercrime also frequently takes the form of illegal gaming, the sale of illegal goods including narcotics and firearms, and the creation, possession, or dissemination of child pornography. It might also involve the illicit global use of remote technologies to steal corporate or governmental secrets. Additionally, cybercrime includes anything from downloading unlawful music to stealing money from online bank accounts [6].

2.3 The classification of cybercrime

The Wall three-category classification system was one of the first reported in academic literature and is therefore often cited. However, the two-category classification system ("cyber-enabled" vs. "cyber-dependent" crime) is the most widely used having been adopted by both researchers and policymakers. Wall's classification scheme, therefore, makes a distinction between [7]:

- "Crimes against the machine," also known as computer integrity crimes, for example, hacking, cracking, and Denial of Service (DoS)/Distributed Denial of Service (DDoS);
- "Crimes using the machine," also known as computer-assisted crimes, for example, piracy, robberies, and scams;
- "Crimes in the machine," also known as computer content crimes, for example, online hate, harassment, and pornography.
- Cybercrime is categorized as follows [8].

2.3.1 Crimes against money

Since the advent of the Internet, most commercial transactions are carried out through this network, such as buying and selling. In the midst of this financial trading, some criminals took advantage of the opportunity to seize them through theft of credit card numbers, illegal electronic transfer of funds, gambling and money laundering, theft and robbery of bank funds, in addition to drug dealing via the Internet.

Financial crimes include a variety of Internet fraud based on so-called "phishing," as well as "Social Engineering" aimed directly at users as well as businesses.

This type of fraud also includes what corrupt employees of financial institutions do by entering wrong data or unauthorized instructions or using unauthorized operations with the aim of stealing, as well as modifying or deleting stored data, or misusing existing system tools, software packages or writing code for fraud purposes.

2.3.2 Crimes against persons

Among the most important of these crimes are:

- The crime of threatening, harassment, and persecution by instilling fear in the soul by pressing the will of the person and intimidating him, as if the perpetrator sends an email to the victim containing frightening and horrific phrases.

- Impersonation, deception, and lure, where the criminal intends to impersonate another person to take advantage of his reputation, for example, his money, his powers, or his influence.

- The manufacture and dissemination of pornography through sites that incite sex for adults and children alike, and these sites publish explicit sexual images of adults and children that can be circulated through various electronic media. The sexual exploitation of children on the Internet takes many forms, from pictures to video recordings of violent sexual crimes.

- Offenses of slander, cursing, and defamation, which are used to harm the honor or dignity and consideration of others. Insults and slander are done through direct lines of communication or be in writing.

2.3.3 Crimes against states

The most notable are:

- Terrorism: At the present time, it has become a global cross-border phenomenon, and the culture of terrorism is broadcast electronically by establishing virtual sites that represent terrorist organizations. Through these sites, they announce their responsibility for one of the attacks that were committed or statements denying that. Terrorist groups also recruit terrorist elements through the Internet. New technologies help them carry out their criminal acts, in addition to publishing visual materials depicting the detention or assassination of the kidnappers.

- Organized crime: This is done where organized crime gangs exploit the available electronic capabilities in planning, passing, and directing criminal schemes and executing and directing criminal operations easily.

- Espionage: In this case, it is intended to see information about the unsecured in another electronic device, and it is not allowed for those who are not authorized to view it, as criminals spy on people, countries, organizations, bodies, or international or national institutions. The espionage crime also includes military espionage, political espionage, and economic espionage.

2.3.4 Crimes against intellectual security

It is through the Internet and various electronic media, cultural, and civilizational attacks that may destabilize the intellectual security of oppressed peoples, and through which the dominant forces spread their thought, language, and values (electronic cultural invasion).

- Electronic warfare: It is already a war between many countries, but through computers and Internet networks, the most prominent example of which was the attack on the infrastructure in Estonia in 2007 by what are believed to be Russian hackers. Analysts believe that this type of attack may become the norm in future wars between countries, where electronic armies will form with the goal of penetrating other countries and destroying their infrastructure, and military leaders may be assigned to lead such wars in the future, and among the most prominent examples of which are currently pirate groups which are called "Syrian Electronic Army," "Iranian Electronic Army," and "Chinese People's Liberation Army Unit" . What can be pointed out is that there are security risks to which information systems are exposed, most notably, viruses, piracy, data fraud, and their use.

According to the 21st note from the National Observatory of Delinquency and Criminal Responses on cybercrime and offenses related to the fraudulent use of the Internet in 2016, Cybercrime can be defined as a set of offenses likely to be committed or facilitated through the use of a computer system, usually connected to a network. Thus defined, it can refer to a wide variety of offenses. Lighting them requires distinguishing between [9]:

- Offenses related to information systems and automated data processing systems originating from the development of computer networks and in particular the Internet. This type of offense means, for example, the alteration of a system, the attack by denial of service, etc.

- Offenses related to "traditional" forms of crime, which may have evolved with new information and communication technologies or been facilitated by them, and therefore constitute a new vector of crime. This second category contains several varieties, including:

- Forms of scams that have emerged with the use of the Internet (fraudulent use of credit cards online, phishing, etc.).

- Threats and insults of any kind disseminated via new means of electronic communication (messaging, forums, social networks, etc.).

- The dissemination of child pornography images facilitated by new communication networks and the Internet.

3. The sexual cybercrime

3.1 Cyberstalking

Cyberstalking is the practice of unwelcome online communication that is persistent. It may involve a variety of incidents, including threats, libel, slander, sexual harassment, or other attempts to intimidate, control, or deceive their victim. A person being stalked online could also be physically followed. It is prohibited in many states and countries, and anyone caught doing it faces criminal prosecution under laws against harassment and stalking or as a designated offense [10].

Cyberstalking has been defined as "the repeated use of the Internet, email, or related digital electronic communication devices to annoy, alarm, or threaten a specific individual." Although some authors, like Bocij et al., describe it as "a totally new form of deviant behavior," it is typically seen as a continuation of more common stalking behaviors that can be carried out through physical presence, telephone, and mail. Perhaps, when viewed objectively, cyberstalking should be seen as a fresh variation on a well-established pattern of criminal behavior, with both similarities and differences to its "terrestrial" cousin. Various commentators, including Koch and Best, have stated that cyberstalking is a "trivial," "rare," or even totally "imaginary" problem. Others, however, contend that internet stalking is becoming more prevalent and that it also has major implications and repercussions for individuals who become victims of it. Because there are relatively few systematic and accurate data from large-scale research, determining the magnitude of cyberstalking occurrences is challenging. We encounter further methodological issues when we consider the various definitions of cyberstalking employed by different analysts, which makes it challenging to cross-compare or aggregate data from multiple analysts. The view of Bocij and McFarlane is more constrained than that of D'Ovidio and Doyle, which covers behaviors that just "annoy," leaving aside the issue of who counts as "reasonable." Therefore, while analyzing the data that is currently accessible, we cannot always be convinced that various measurements of cyberstalking activities are founded upon the same or similar notions of what constitutes appropriate behavior. Nevertheless, we can take note of analyses and projections that provide a general sense of how pervasive a cyberstalking problem may actually be [11].

The Internet gives stalkers the chance to bother their targets while pretending to be anonymous. "The repeated use of the Internet, email, or related digital electronic communication means to annoy, scare, or threaten a particular individual or group of individuals" is the definition of cyberstalking. All 50 States and the federal government have passed laws intended to protect victims of cyberstalking since this crime has grown so pervasive. In a study WHO analyze 201 closed cases of aggravated harassment between January 1996 and August 2000 that were investigated by the New York Police Department's Computer Investigation and Technology Unit (CITU). The majority of the offenders in these cases were men (80%), 74% of whom were White, 13% Asian, 8% Hispanic, and 5% Black. Although 26% of these offenders were minors, the average age of the cyberstalkers was 24. Females made up 52% of the victims of cyberstalking, although many of the targets were institutions including universities, businesses, and government organizations. The victims comprised 85% White people, 6% Asian people, 5% Black people, and 4% Hispanic people. The victims were 32 on average. The majority of cases (92%) solely employed one type of technology. In 79% of the cases, email was utilized, and in 13% of the cases, instant messaging was used. The difficulties that law enforcement encounters while handling cyberstalking cases are also covered by the authors. The two biggest obstacles to obtaining account data and user information from Internet service providers are stated as jurisdictional problems and privacy problems. The growing use of technology and the anonymity of cyberstalking will probably continue to drive up the rate of this kind of crime [12].

How technology is misused in cases of sexual assault, cyberbullying, or stalking, as well as domestic violence Here is a research scenario that uses specific abuse strategies and dynamics to show how abusers exert power and influence over victims, particularly women [13]:

Sentimental or meaty abuse: Situations that put down the use of technology may develop into this form of abuse. Using technology to portray you as dependent on it or as a threat.

Disjunction: The abuser discovers the victim's secret location. Use technology to ruin both your personal and professional reputation. Unwanted emails or texts tend to be abusive or pornographic in nature.

Criminal force or threat: The abuser discovers the victim's secret location. Use technology to ruin both your personal and professional reputation. Unwanted emails or texts tend to be abusive or pornographic in nature.

Abusage in the context of profitability: This type of abuse is happening more frequently by impersonating or following profitable online financial accounts. By impersonating fraudulent activity, it can lower your credit and loan ratings.

Using advantage and unjust treatment: By seeming to be something to make you feel foolish, incapable of understanding things readily, or wary of technology, it performs a very important function.

Taking advantage of others: This abuse can be used as an optional category by preying on others, such as children, friends, or family members, to annoy them and set up devices to obtain information about their account information through the use of technology.

Stalking or bullying and Intimidating: And finally, one type of abuse involves employing technology to observe or report. Diminishing technology or referring to gadgets by secretly altering information or device settings Constant contact with you could be another form of abuse that is minimized, denied, or blamed.

3.2 Child sexual abuse material

In the official INHOPE website specializing in child protection, it is mentioned that Child Sexual Abuse Material (CSAM) has different legal definitions in different countries. The minimum defines CSAM as imagery or videos which show a person who is a child and engaged in or is depicted as being engaged in explicit sexual activity.

Sometimes CSAM is referred to as child pornography. However, the term "child pornography" should be avoided for the following reasons:

The term child pornography fails to convey the content's true nature and downplays how serious the abuse is from the child's point of view.

The term "pornography" is typically used to refer to content that is distributed for the aim of evoking sexual pleasure and showing consenting persons in sexual activity. Using this phrase in relation to kids has the risk of normalizing, trivializing, and even legitimizing child sexual abuse and exploitation.

Kid pornography implies consent, which a child is unable to offer in a legal sense. The term child pornography is still used in legislation in some countries. For this reason, CSAM is sometimes referred to as child pornography for legal purposes.
In non-legal contexts, such as in media publications, the term Child Sexual Abuse Material (CSAM) should be used.

One of the issues that cause disagreement is the age of consent to sexual relations. For this reason, the age at which an individual is considered a child differs from country to country.

Legislation also differs in regard to images of children who have been instructed to pose in sexualised ways. In many countries, images and videos of children who are completely or partially undressed and in sexualized poses, and images which are focused on children's sexual organs are also illegal and should be reported to your national hotline. A further area where legislation differs is whether an actual child has to be depicted in the image, or whether artificially created images constitute CSAM. The legal sanctions for production, distribution, and possession of CSAM also differ from country to country [14].

Child sexual abuse material is obtained and shared in several ways:

- The sexual abuse of a child is caught on camera by the predator, who subsequently uploads or spreads it online.

- Through an app or service on a connected device, a predator makes contact with a youngster and tricks or coerces them into creating and distributing sexually explicit photographs and videos of themselves. This is encouraged by predators who manipulate and threaten children while "grooming" them to trust them. A predator shares images or videos of children "stolen" from social media accounts.

Online child sex abuse material is sold all over the world and is repulsive. Demand for fresh and more violent material is increased every time a picture or video of a child being molested is uploaded or spread [15].

3.3 Sexual solicitation

The Internet provides young persons with abundant possibilities while also increasing their exposure to risks, such as being solicited for sexual purposes. Online sexual solicitation concerns acts "of encouraging someone to talk about sex, to do something sexual, or to share personal sexual information." The effects on victims have been shown to include anxiety, post-traumatic stress disorder, depression, and developmental disruption.

The Internet is an integral part of everyday life activities. The upsurge of routine Internet use among youth affords solicitation offenders an unlimited source of potential victims at any time or place, while capable guardians are often lacking online. As routine activity theory postulates, crime rates increase when suitable targets, absent guardians, and motivated offenders converge. This has been applied effectively to various forms of cybercrime, such as fraud or bullying. Plausibly, the Internet may also provide an ideal criminogenic context for sexual solicitation of minors [16].

3.4 Sextortion

Sextortion is actually defined differently by different people. There are two widely used definitions of sextortion: (1) sextortion is when a perpetrator threatens to share a victim's private sexual images in order to extort something from them or (2) sextortion is when a victim is coerced into sending sexual material to the perpetrator, either through the threat of sharing private sexual images or some other threat of harm. Depending on whether the culprit must genuinely own the photographs or can only claim to own the images, the initial view can have a different scope. Scholars, the media, and the general public occasionally mix up sextortion and revenge porn, but even though these crimes are frequently associated, they must be distinguished from one another. The nonconsensual sharing of a victim's pornographic material is known as "revenge porn," a term that is less widely used but more appropriately described as "nonconsensual porn." Because sextortion frequently involves the threat of retaliatory pornography against a victim unless they comply with demands made of them, this relationship between the two crimes contributes to their confusion. Both sextortion and revenge porn are sex-related cybercrimes, however, unlike revenge porn, sextortion relies heavily on coerced quiet to succeed. The goal of sextortion is typically to gain sexual material or money, and the victim's silence and fear of embarrassment are vital to attaining that goal. Therefore, even if the sextortionist has access to the victim's private information, they will not necessarily publicize it. In contrast, the goal of revenge porn is to disseminate the victim's sexually explicit content, and the victim's silence does not significantly hinder this goal from being accomplished [17].

3.5 Grooming

According to the definition of child sexual grooming, it is "a communication process by which a perpetrator uses affinity seeking strategies, while concurrently engaging in sexual desensitization and gathering information about targeted victims with the aim to develop relationships that result in need fulfillment, such as physical sexual solicitation." Therefore, the labels "pedophile" or "sexual predator" are frequently used to refer to such individuals [18].

Grooming, or pedotrapage, refers to the solicitation of children for sexual purposes by a stranger or an acquaintance, its psychological manipulation. If this practice occurs mainly on the Internet, it can also take place in everyday life. Concretely, the offender will first do everything to put the child in trust to create an emotional relation with him. He will make sure to gradually separate him from his family and friends in order to create a feeling of dependence in him. Grooming can take different forms. It generally results in the purchase of gifts, compliments, the sharing of secrets, a benevolent listening. In a way, the offender takes on the role of "protector." If the attack takes place online, the offender may ask the child for pornographic photos, including pretending to be someone his own age and he can use these to blackmail him or to distribute them on the Internet. The offender does not always intend to meet the young person in person to "take action." The problem is that the child is not aware of the harmful nature of this relationship [19].

3.6 Cybersex trafficing

The live online sexual exploitation of children is known as "cybersex trafficking." Nowadays, predators and pedophiles can conduct searches online and wire a secure payment to an adult who organizes the event. Children as young as 2 years old are subjected to maltreatment or forced to engage in sex activities in front of webcams. The customer pays more the more abusive the show is. Cybersex trafficking victims can be relocated to and mistreated everywhere there is an internet connection, a webcam, or even just a cell phone, unlike victims of bars or brothels with a fixed address. Trafficking in virtual sex has developed into a lucrative cottage industry that is frightening [20].

3.7 Cybersex tourism

According to the United Nations World Tourism Organization, "trips organized from within the sector, or from outside this sector but using its structures and networks with the primary purpose of effecting a commercial sexual relationship by the tourist with the residents at the destination," are considered sex tourism. As a result, sex tourism is an activity that involves people traveling domestically and internationally to engage in sexual activity that is both against the law and unethical for them. Sex tourism is regarded as one of the top five largest illicit and criminal activity-involved enterprises in the world. Sex tourism includes both human trafficking, including the sale of men, women, and even children, in addition to travel arrangements made particularly for sex or novel sexual encounters for clients. Involvement in forced labor and commercial sexual servitude affects over 20.9 million people and children globally [21].

Growingly more people are using the Internet, which has made it easier to exploit minors live via new technology. The International Union of the United Nations Telecommunications predicts that by the end of 2014, there will be 3 billion Internet users, with two-thirds coming from poorer nations. New behaviors are produced by these technological advancements, such as webcam child sex tourism (WCST). Additionally, globalization has boosted cross-cultural interactions, uniting many communities. Another element that encourages child commercial sexual exploitation is poverty. Due to the financial crisis, many people have turned to being exploited or becoming exploiters in order to make money. Financially unstable times also result in court system instability, which breeds corruption and makes it more challenging to bring offenders to justice [22].

3.8 Sexting

Sexting has developed as a result of the easy accessibility of mobile communication technology and the rise in internet usage. Using mobile devices or the Internet to send or upload sexually explicit text messages and images, including nude or semi-naked photos, is known as sexting. When the photographs from "sexting" are released without the victim's knowledge, it becomes an issue and is considered a kind of cybercrime. This may occur by "hacking," in which the photographs are taken from the intended recipient without their permission, or it may occur when the intended receiver shares the images (with friends, on internet forums, etc.) without the sender's knowledge. Senders may be ignorant that their photographs may be distributed, or a previously trusted recipient may be unworthy of that trust (e.g., an ex-partner who shares images; this is commonly referred to as "revenge pornography"). According to research, women only typically send sexual photographs in the context of relationships where there is trust; as a result, the sender has little reason to believe that the images will be shared without their knowledge at the time they are sent. However, because the photographs uploaded online are permanent, the damage is ongoing and intensified. Even if the original pictures or movies are taken down, duplicates may still exist and be shared forever. Since the victim's reputation could be permanently damaged on both a personal and professional level, the long-term effects of such a crime may be much more detrimental than they were intended to be [23].

4. The transition from sexual cybercrime to physical assault

Sexual, psychological, or emotional abuse of women online is also common. It has the ability to cause abuse and violence offline, as well as bodily harm. The same tendencies exist both online and offline; for instance, technology makes intimate partner violence more prevalent online. Because of this, it is impossible to separate online abuse and violence against women from what occurs offline; both online and offline locations can become the scene of such behavior. Women's abuse and violence online must be considered a form of physical abuse and violence [24].

Cyberviolence can cause enormous damage to victims and often precedes episodes of physical violence or even homicide, especially in the context of separation [25].

Physical violence against women may occur simultaneously with, aggravate, or be caused by cyberviolence. The 23-year-old Pennsylvania guy waited outside her house with a boxcutter and a revolver after his Facebook threats to get his ex-partner to return by posting sexual photographs of her failed. Similarly, a 31-year-old woman in Seattle who was the target of revenge porn while being cyberstalked by her ex-police partner was choked and knocked to the ground during a physical altercation with him. 3.3% of women experienced physical abuse that was made worse by online violence, whereas 5% of women suffered bodily hurt and abuse as a result of online violence. A significant percentage of women (12%) also mentioned getting sick physically as a result of violence [26].

An example of cyberbullying which was represented by the newspaper named Le Parisien which reports the suffering of a young girl from the suburbs of Rouen (Seine-Maritime) on the verge of suicide who had filed a complaint in November 2015 against an Internet user who demanded a sexual relationship her under penalty of sharing on the Internet all her photos if she refuses his request [27].

So cybersex crime can go from harassment on the internet to the risk of real sexual assault, especially if the victim does not file a complaint against the cyber offender and submits to his demands. The very vulnerable position of the victim is explained by the fact of the feeling of shame and fear.

Blackmail, in particular through cyber-harassment, can be considered an aggravating circumstance of physical or sexual assault.

Children who have WCST may suffer exceedingly dire outcomes. First off, victims of sexual abuse and assault may experience a wide range of physical consequences, including genital injury, deformities, unintended pregnancies, and an increased risk of catching the AIDS virus. Even when there is no direct interaction between the abuser and the victim in TSW, the child may nonetheless experience abuse from middlemen. Sexual abuse can also result in a variety of psychological problems. Indicators of hostility, anxiety, and depression are seen in children from WCST. The psychological effects of sexual abuse may also include remorse, anxiety, and low self-esteem. As a result of these long-lasting psychological impacts, which may also result in nightmares, suicidal, anorexic, or other physically dangerous inclinations, the child's health will be permanently impacted. Additionally, photos of child pornography created and spread by modern technologies never fully vanish from the Internet, which has especially negative effects on the child because there may be a sensation of abuse with each new viewing. In terms of their social development, children who have trouble trusting adults run the danger of isolating themselves or acting aggressively, which hinders their ability to build relationships with others.

In order for governments to effectively address emerging problems like WCST, the reintegration of juvenile victims of commercial sexual exploitation must continue to be a top priority [22].

Sex tourism leads in both the infringement of human rights and freedoms as well as the exploitation of people. On a national and worldwide scale, studies have shown that sex tourism contributes to the spread of teen pregnancy as well as the so-called sexually transmitted illnesses. The development of mental and emotional illnesses in its victims, such as substance misuse, depression, and suicide, is also attributed to sex tourism [21].

A technique known as grooming involves an adult purposefully approaching kids and controlling them for sex. The groomers try to establish a relationship of trust with the child by showing interest, giving compliments in order to gradually lead him to questions and acts with a sexual connotation. Grooming can lead to sexual violence online (via webcam, chat, email, etc.) or in real life (via physical encounter). In addition, the groomer can create or spread images, which makes the child again a victim. In this setting, the culprit tries to limit his own risks by revealing as little as possible about himself. He also encourages the child not to talk about their friendship under the guise of "our little secret" [28]. The purpose of the physical encounter is not necessarily immediate sexual contact, but sometimes it requires a new period of socialization before the criminal act [29].

Another consequence, once the predator and the child have formed a bond, the predator may start introducing the youngster to pornography and then recommend taking pictures of the child in a sexually suggestive position. This procedure aims to desensitize the child to nudity, pique their interest in sex, and normalize adult–child sexual interactions [30].

In an odd instance, the accuser was found guilty of rape without physical contact after coercing a 15-year-old girl into engaging in sexual self-penetration. Without any consent during a webcam conversation, after he threatened to spread compromising photos. The presiding judge in the case considered such an act of raping, stating that even though there was no physical contact. There was no consent and he manipulated the youngster through real blackmail, so he forced her to digitally penetrate herself [31].

A study on forensic intelligence-led prevention of drug-facilitated sexual assaults applies information from both criminology and forensic science, and it encourages interdisciplinary discussion between the two fields. These days, there are not many initiatives that support this interdisciplinary conversation between forensic science and criminology. This framework serves two purposes: it may be used as a research tool to gather forensic and criminological data in order to comprehend a criminal phenomenon and it can serve as a platform for strategic thought and action in order to combat it. In a similar vein, additional approaches suggested for promoting interdisciplinary interaction between forensic science and criminology also collect and evaluate pertinent data from both fields regarding a particular crime occurrence to later produce well-targeted, evidence-based preventive measures [32].

Finally, in my opinion as a forensic pathologist, it emerges from this general analysis that cybercrime against people, particularly of a sexual nature, has a major impact on the real lives of victims, whether through physical aggression at the origin of bodily injuries, sexual assault or even disabling psychological damage or sexually transmitted diseases. the transition from online virtual aggression to aggression in real life is obvious and the risk is major especially if the victim is a child because he does not have the consent nor the discernment to judge his relationships and the extent of the risks of his environment. Cybersex crimes attract victims to lose their decision-making control because of the shame and harassing pressure imposed by the aggressor and they can responding to the claims of the aggressors or entering into a conflict that generates violence and physical harm to the victims. Moreover, in order to combat the phenomenon of sexual cybercrime, a partnership between forensic medicine and cybersecurity is urgently advised.

5. Conclusion

Sexual cybercrime is a scourge that can ravage our society if we do not react against crime in cyber space and particularly against cybersex crime, which mainly targets young women and children.

The transition from the virtual form of sexual cybercrime to the form of real physical (bodily and psychological) assault is often a predictable and very dangerous development with serious harm to the victims.

The obligation to fight against this social scourge has imposed the development of cyber security as well as the establishment of legislative texts devoted to the protection of cybercrime and particularly of the sexual type.

Conflict of Interest

The authors declare no conflict of interest.

Author details

Mohammed Hedidi
Public Hospital Establishment of Timimoun, Timimoun, Algeria

*Address all correspondence to: hedidisoft@hotmail.fr

References

[1] Sunil CP, Mente RS, Chendage BD. Cyber crime, cyber space and effects of cyber crime. International Journal of Scientific Research in Computer Science, Engineering and Information Technology. 2021;**7**:210-214. DOI: 10.32628/CSEIT217139

[2] HuanGuo Z, WenBao H, XueJia L, DongDai L, JianFeng M, JianHua L. Survey on cyberspace security. Science China Information Sciences. 2015;**58**:1-43. DOI: 10.1007/s11432-015-5433-4

[3] Burden K, Palmer C. Cyber crime – A new breed of criminal? Computer Law and Security Review. 2003;**19**:222. DOI: 10.1016/s0267-3649(03)00306-6

[4] Tsakalidis G, Vergidis K. A systematic approach toward description and classification of cybercrime incidents. IEEE Transactions on Systems, Man, and Cybernetics: Systems. 2017;**49**:710-729. DOI: 10.1109/TSMC.2017.2700495

[5] Council of Europe. Convention on cybercrime. European Treaty Series No. 185; Council of Europe: Budapest, Hungary, 2001; pp. 1-25. Available from: https://rm.coe.int/1680081561. [Accessed: September 4, 2022]

[6] Deora RS, Chudasama D. Brief study of cybercrime on an internet. Journal of Communication Engineering & Systems. 2021;**11**:2-3. DOI: 10.37591/JoCES

[7] Phillips K, Davidson JC, Farr RR, Burkhardt C, Caneppele S, Aiken MP. Conceptualizing cybercrime: Definitions, typologies and taxonomies. Forensic Science. 2022;**2**(2):379-398. DOI: 10.3390/forensicsci2020028

[8] Rezki K. Cyberspace and cyber crime –towards modeling behavior and controlling action. Journal of Human Sciences, Oum El Bouaghi University. 2022;**9**:597-609 ISSN 1112-9255/E-ISSN 2588-2414

[9] L'Observatoire national de la délinquance et des réponses pénales (ONDRP), La cybercriminalité et les infractions liées à l'utilisation frauduleuse d'internet en 2016: éléments de mesure et d'analyse, N°21. [Internet]. 2017 [cited 2017 Nov]. Available from: https://www.ihemi.fr/sites/default/files/publications/files/2019-12/note_21_0.pdf. [Accessed: September 7, 2022]

[10] Sammons J, Cross M, editors. Beyond technology-dealing with people. The Basics of Cyber Safety Computer and Mobile Device Safety Made Easy. 1st ed. Cambridge. 2017. pp. 179-200. DOI: 10.1016/ B978-0-12-416650-9.00009-7

[11] Majid Y, editor. Cyberstalking. In: Cybercrime and Society. 1st ed. London; 2006. pp. 127-130. DOI: /10.4135/9781446212196

[12] Robert D'Ovidio MS, Doyle J. Study on cyberstalking: Understanding investigative hurdles. FBI Law Enforcement Bulletin. 2003;**72**:10-17 NCJ Number: 199743

[13] Chahal R, Kumar L, Jindal S, Rawat P. Cyber stalking: Technological form of sexual harassment. International Journal on Emerging Technologies. 2019;**10**:367-373. DOI: 10.13140/RG.2.2.27772.90246

[14] INHOPE. What is child sexual abuse material? [Internet]. 2021 [2021 Jan 04]. Available from: https://www.inhope.org/EN/articles/child-sexual-abuse-material?locale=en. [Accessed: September 8, 2022]

[15] eSafety Commissioner. Child sexual abuse material [internet]. 2020 [2020 Mar]. Available from: https://crimestoppers.com.au/wp/wp-content/uploads/2020/03/CS-eSafety-Fact-Sheet-Child-Sexual-Abuse-Material.pdf. [Accessed: September 8, 2022]

[16] Schulz A, Bergen E, Schuhmann P, Hoyer J¨r, Santtila P. Online sexual solicitation of minors: How often and between whom does it occur? Journal of Research in Crime and Delinquency. 2016;**52**:165-188. DOI: 10.1177/0022427815599426

[17] Carlton A. Sextortion: The hybrid "cyber-sex" crime. North Carolina Journal of Law & Technology. 2020;**21**:178-214 Available from: https://scholarship.law.unc.edu/ncjolt/vol21/iss3/5. [Accessed: September 9, 2022]

[18] C.H Ngejane, J.H.P Eloff, G Mabuza-Hocquet, Mitigating online sexual grooming cybercrime on social media using machine learning: A desktop survey. In: International Conference on Advances in Big Data, Computing and Data Communication Systems (icABCD) ; 6-7 August 2018 ; Durban, South Africa: IEEE;2018. DOI: 10.1109/ICABCD.2018.8465413

[19] Julie Giorgetta. Le grooming: cette pratique dangereuse pour nos enfants [internet], 2021[2021 Dec 07]. Available from: https://www.passeportsante.net/famille/adolescence?doc=grooming-cette-pratique-dangereuse-nos-enfants. [Accessed: September 9, 2022]

[20] IJM Casework Series. Cybersex trafficking [Internet]. 2019. Available from: https://ijmstoragelive.blob.core.windows.net/ijmna/documents/IJM-2019-Casework_FactSheets_CSEC.pdf. [Accessed: September 10, 2022]

[21] Commission of Crime Prevention and Criminal Justice. LASALLEMUN 2018 "Stop wishing, start doing" background guide [Internet]. 2018. Available from: http://lasallecancun.edu.mx/lasallemun/wp-content/uploads/2018/02/BG-CCPCJ.pdf. [Accessed: September 11, 2022]

[22] End Child Prostitution, Child Pornography and Trafficking of Children for Sexual Purposes. Webcam child sex tourism [Internet]. 2014. Available from: https://ecpat.be/wp-content/uploads/2017/12/webcam-english2.pdf. [Accessed: September 11, 2022]

[23] The Open University, The Psychology of Cybercrime, Sexting [Internet]. Available from: https://www.open.edu/openlearn/health-sports-psychology/psychology/the-psychology-cybercrime/content-section-2.2.1. [Accessed: September 11, 2022]

[24] Maria Vlahakis. Womankind worldwide, breaking the silence: Ending online violence and abuse against women's rights activists [Internet]. 2018. Available from: https://www.womankind.org.uk/wp-content/uploads/2020/08/breaking-the-silence-policy-briefing.pdf. [Accessed: September 11, 2022]

[25] Mylène Fernet. Cyber violence conjugale et séparation: une synthèse des connaissances pour mieux comprendre le phénomène et orienter les actions [Internet]. 2018. Available from: https://frq.gouv.qc.ca/en/story-and-report/intimate-partner-cyber-violence-and-separation-a-knowledge-synthesis-to-better-understand-the-phenomenon-and-guide-actions/. [Accessed September 11, 2022]

[26] Jessica West. Cyber-violence against women prepared for battered women's support services [Internet]. 2014. Available from: https://www.bwss.org/wp-content/uploads/2014/05/

CyberVAWReportJessicaWest.pdf. [Accessed: September 11, 2022]

[27] Frédéric Naizot. Garges: l'étudiant se livrait au chantage sexuel sur Internet [Internet]. 2017. Available from: https://www.leparisien.fr/val-d-oise-95/garges-les-gonesse-95140/garges-l-etudiant-condamne-pour-s-etre-livre-au-chantage-sexuel-sur-internet-03-01-2017-6521238.php. [Accessed: September 11, 2020]

[28] Sécurité en ligne, Parents [internet]. 2022. Available from: https://childfocus.be/fr be/S%C3%A9curit%C3%A9-en-ligne/Parents. [Accessed: September 11, 2022]

[29] Aude Ventéjoux. Une lecture de la cyberviolence: la rencontre du sujet et du cyberespace dans les infractions à caractère sexuel envers mineurs réalisées sur Internet [thesis]. Université Rennes 2 UFR Sciences Sociales, Pl. Recteur Henri le Moal, 35000 Rennes, France; 2019

[30] Ilene R. Berson, grooming cybervictims: The psychosocial effects of online exploitation for youth. Journal of School Violence. 2008;**2**:5-8. DOI: 10.1300/J202v02n01_02

[31] Paris Match. Cyber-harcèlement: Un Belge reconnu coupable de viol « à distance »[Internet]. 2018. Available from: https://parismatch.be/actualites/societe/177784/cyber-harcelement-un-belge-reconnu-coupable-de-viol-a-distance. [Accessed: September 11, 2022]

[32] Prego-Meleiro P, García-Ruiz C, Sanz-Pareja M, Esnoz IR, Quintanilla MG, Montalvo G. Forensic intelligence-led prevention of drug-facilitated sexual assaults. Forensic Science International. 2022;**337**:1-11. DOI: 10.1016/j.forsciint.2022.111373